HORMONE POWER

MARJOLEIN DUBBERS

HORMONE POWER

Transform Your Diet,
Transform Your Life

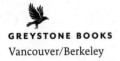

GREYSTONE BOOKS
Vancouver/Berkeley

19 20 21 22 23   5 4 3 2 1

Greystone Books Ltd.
greystonebooks.com

Cataloguing data available from Library and Archives Canada
ISBN 978-1-77164-355-9 (pbk.)
ISBN 978-1-77164-356-6 (ePub)

Editing by Stephanie Fysh
Cover image by Saskia Lelieveld
Cover design by Briana Garelli and Nayeli Jimenez
Interior design by Nayeli Jimenez
Typesetting by Shed Simas/Onça Design
Printed and bound in Canada on ancient-forest-friendly paper by Friesens

Greystone Books gratefully acknowledges the Musqueam, Squamish, and Tsleil-Waututh peoples on whose land our office is located.

Greystone Books thanks the Canada Council for the Arts, the British Columbia Arts Council, the Province of British Columbia through the Book Publishing Tax Credit, and the Government of Canada for supporting our publishing activities.

Canada

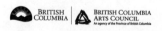

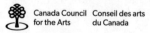

The advice provided in this book has been carefully considered and checked by the author and publisher. It should not, however, be regarded as a substitute for competent medical advice. Therefore, all information in this book is provided without any warranty or guarantee on the part of the publisher or the author. Neither the author nor the publisher or their representatives shall bear any liability whatsoever for personal injury, property damage, and financial losses.

CONTENTS

The food you eat can be either the safest and most powerful form of medicine or the slowest form of poison.

ANN WIGMORE

———————————————

To all women who take the responsibility for their physical and mental health into their own hands

INTRODUCTION

WHEN I TURNED 52, my body gave me a wonderful gift: I ended up totally burned out. Of course, at the time I didn't see it as a gift—it was a problem or a failure, as much a failure of my body as myself. Even though I felt completely done in, the only thing I wanted was to quickly return to my more-than-full-time workweek, with long commutes, draining meetings, and workplace stress, but also with great colleagues and the good feeling that I was involved in tasks with purpose.

"MA'AM, WHAT MORE DO YOU ACTUALLY WANT?"

Because I was in reasonably good shape, I thought I'd recover quickly, but in that I was bitterly disappointed. To be honest, I knew that my condition had declined over the previous year. A year before that I'd gone to my family doctor with complaints about exhaustion and my diminished strength as a runner. Blood work showed nothing out of the ordinary. That summer, for the first time, I didn't fit into my cute white summer slacks, even though my diet and fitness regime hadn't changed. It was *very* frustrating.

Given that my issues had gotten worse, I was referred to a neurologist. He also couldn't find anything. His message was "Ma'am, you're over 50. It's normal to lose some muscle strength, be able to do less, and feel tired more quickly." To me it sounded like "Ma'am, you're 50—what *more* do you actually want?"

I had accepted his statement, but now, at home on leave due to burnout, his words came back to me. Was I really in the autumn of my life? Were the best years of my life behind me? If I were to believe everyone who speaks or writes on this topic, a woman over 50 is past her prime. After 40 it's all downhill: memory, muscle strength, hormones, healthy hair, concentration, metabolism, and let's not forget, libido—in short, our overall vitality and health. Everything decreases, with one exception: our spare tire. That's also out of balance, but it's on the road to getting bigger.

AUTUMN? ALREADY?

Books about menopause talk about the "autumn of our days" and the "wisdom of the ripe woman." To be honest, I didn't understand that at all. I didn't feel like it was my season for harvest, and more often than not, I didn't feel ripe or wise. In fact, I still wanted to be seeding all sorts of new things in my life, although I wasn't quite sure what. I had the feeling that there was still so much I wanted to do and *could* do that I just hadn't quite got to because I'd been so busy with my work. But if my vitality and health were only going to decline, then I had a big problem. My life would be over long before I felt like I'd lived it. Could that really be the way things were going to be?

I still remember this feeling of despair as if it were yesterday— that feeling that while I was definitely over 50, I still hadn't lived the life I wanted. To be honest, I often thought my real life had yet to begin, that I was still standing in the starter blocks.

I suddenly realized that I'd always been busy with other people's goals. In particular, a large part of my life, over 25 years, had been dedicated to my employers. What were *my* goals? What did I want? All of a sudden I felt it was urgent to get my life back on the right road.

STRAIN UPON STRAIN UPON STRAIN

On the internet, I searched for what exactly was wrong with me and what I needed to fix it. I read that if you always demand too much of yourself, you can end up burned out, and I learned that as a result my adrenal glands had become exhausted. Adrenal glands are the organs that work overtime if they think you're in danger. Draining meetings and other work-related stress acted as alarms for my adrenal glands. Who would have thought?

I also discovered that as a woman in menopause, my adrenal glands were especially vulnerable, because during this time they have added responsibilities. They have to take over the ovaries' job of producing estrogen and progesterone. But if there is too much stress, the adrenal glands just don't get around to that, and a shortage of estrogen and progesterone results in an avalanche of other problems, among them an underactive thyroid, due to which you can feel dog-tired. Do you see the pattern? In short, experiencing too much stress during menopause became a strain on top of a strain on top of another strain. So now what? I learned that for women all hormones are complexly intertwined and more or less determine everything about your vitality and health. How could I give them a helping hand? What did my hormones need?

MALNOURISHED? *ME?*

I began to deepen my understanding of hormones and nutrition and came to the shocking conclusion that I was malnourished. Not that I had such a bad diet, but it simply wasn't nutritious enough for a 50+ woman in our hectic society.

Often my breakfast was yogurt with some crispy granola (healthy, right?); my lunch was soup and salad at the office (also not so bad... was it?); I wasn't a snacker, just some fruit around four o'clock. But my dinner sometimes was a bust. I'd lived alone for years, so nobody was at home waiting for me. The various train stations along my commute regularly provided me with something that served as dinner. This could be coffee with a cheese croissant, or some fruit juice and a bag of M&Ms. Luckily, I often had dinner parties with colleagues and friends, and made up for the damage by eating a lot of vegetables…or so I thought. In fact, I didn't at all.

Once I learned how many and which vitamins and minerals a woman's body needs to function properly, and where those nutrients can be found (and, most critically, where you won't find them), I could come to no other conclusion than that I was severely malnourished, probably had been for years. No wonder my body was putting me on notice!

....

I came to the conclusion that the biggest gains
to be made were in the realm of nutrition.

....

I concluded that I could improve my diet. I bought a blender and learned how to make green smoothies. I discovered an urban organic farm in my neighborhood and visited a health food store where I encountered new products such as quinoa and hempseed. I took a course about raw food, bought a juicer, and visited what was at that time the only store in Amsterdam that specialized in superfoods.

As my energy levels rose, so too did the pile of related books on my bookshelves, and I went from one astonishment to the other. Nutrition appeared to be so much more than just what I put in my mouth. The pinnacle of my astonishment was my meeting with Ruth.

RUTH'S STORY

I first encountered Ruth Heidrich telling her life story in a YouTube video. Just like me, she loved running and thought that she lived a healthy life, but when she was 47 Ruth learned she had breast cancer. After surgery she radically changed her diet and began to dream of participating in a triathlon: a 3.8-kilometer swim, a 180-kilometer bike ride, and a marathon. Two years later she participated in the Ironman in Hawaii, one of the most challenging triathlons in the world, and proudly crossed the finish line. After that came many more triathlons and competitions, after she turned 50, then after 60, and even well into her 70s!

I suddenly realized that it was possible—that a woman's body in its 70s *could* still be able to do a triathlon. Wow! It's not preordained that a woman goes downhill after 40. She can also climb to a peak! What do you mean, there's only harvesting after 50? There's still lots of time to sow!

HORMONE BALANCE THROUGH DIET

After several months of healthy eating, other aspects of a healthy lifestyle such as rest and exercise, and watching inspirational talks, I slowly transformed from a lump on the couch into a woman with a mission. With my increased energy, my dream became to tell other women that there's so much more life to be lived if you start to feed yourself properly—that life doesn't have to be put in neutral but can be lived at full throttle. And I wanted to show that good nutrition is something quite different from what we've been raised to believe is good for us.

It wasn't just that I had more energy. Issues I'd struggled with so long that I barely noticed them anymore disappeared. The painful arthritis in my fingers, for example, which my mother and grandmother also had. The uncontrollable food cravings. Cellulitis, which I'd long ago accepted as inevitable, mostly disappeared. My hair was thicker and my nails no longer broke. I felt like running again, and people started telling me how good I looked. Without fully realizing it, I had eaten my way back to balanced hormones. I lived it, and I believed it, but still I was surprised. Was even *more* possible?

CHANGE YOUR DIET. CHANGE YOUR HORMONES. CHANGE YOUR LIFE.

Since that realization a lot has happened: I finally pulled away from the starting line of my life. I trained to become a vitality coach, resigned from my job, started my private practice, founded the Energetic Women's Academy, and built my online presence. I developed the online program The Energetic Woman's Nutrition Compass and was able to guide thousands of women toward greater health and vitality, so that they could make their own dreams come true. My desire to share my knowledge with even more women has only become stronger—hence this book.

I hope you will use the insights and ideas you find here to improve the quality of *your* life. An energized body can give you the life you dearly want, regardless of how old you are. In Part 1 you will read about the most important hormones in your body and how they work together. I explain which symptoms are associated with certain hormonal imbalances, and I give you tips that you can start using today.

In Part 2 you'll read about the seven key principles of the Nutrition Compass, because of course you'll want more than just the initial tips. If you follow all the key principles of the Nutrition Compass, your hormones will become balanced, you'll be full of energy, your ailments will disappear, and you'll have an easier time achieving a healthy weight.

Throughout the book I've sprinkled my favorite recipes—the tastiest and especially the easiest. It might be that you aren't yet familiar with some of the ingredients. Take a chance: buy one or two and start experimenting. Many are available online, so you don't even need to leave your house.

THE KEY IS IN YOUR HANDS

I'm convinced that if more women make their dreams come true, the world will be a better place. So many women never realize their beautiful dreams because they have minimal energy and stamina and aren't healthy enough. I don't like the word "must," but now I'll use it: This must change! When it comes to your health, the time has passed for relying on others. The key is in *your* hands. This is very much in your control. You will understand how good nutrition can improve your life only when you've experienced it. Change your diet and give it a try. I promise you—you can do more than you think! If I can do it, you can too. No matter how old you are, make sure you're fit enough for the future that awaits you, and make your dreams come true. Every journey begins with the first step. Are you coming?

HOMEMADE NONDAIRY MILK

I want to encourage you to make your own nondairy milk. It's tastier, cheaper, and especially much healthier than those expensive supermarket cartons of nondairy milk, which are mostly water, their healthy ingredients diminished by processing and packaging. For this recipe, use raw nuts and seeds. My favorite ingredients for nondairy milk are almonds, cashews, pumpkin seeds, and rolled oats.

Nuts and seeds provide zinc, magnesium, selenium, and the important B vitamins that give you energy. Walnuts provide healthy omega-3 fatty acids. Unfortunately, oats, nuts, and seeds do contain phytic acid, which can impede your intestines' absorption of vitamins and minerals. You can improve their nutritional benefits by soaking them overnight to reduce the phytic acid.

Here's What You Need

1 cup raw nuts or seeds
cheesecloth or a fine sieve that tapers to a point

Here's How You Make It

Soak the raw nuts or seeds overnight. Drain them and rinse. Place them in your blender with 5 cups of water. Blend thoroughly. Pour the mixture through the cheesecloth or fine sieve. (A sieve with a tapered end makes this very easy.) Store the nondairy milk in the fridge in a glass jar or bottle. It will last for 5 days. You can use your nondairy milk in smoothies, breakfasts, dressings, and desserts.

PART ONE

Hormones: The Key to Vitality and Health

1

WOMEN REALLY
ARE DIFFERENT

M Y PARENTS HAD seven daughters and no sons. One day my father teased my six sisters and me by saying that he tried to have *eleven* sons, because then he would have had his own soccer team, but after seven girls in a row he gave up hope. We got him back by saying that it didn't seem *that* difficult to just add that "extra piece" that makes a boy.

HAVE YOU EVER SEEN A HORMONE?

The difference between men and women is, of course, not just that "extra piece" boys are born with. Men and women are exponentially different. Nature has designed women for the most amazing of Earth's wonders: we can create a new life. This is why a woman's body is so different from a man's, and why those differences are much deeper than just how we look on the outside. The biggest difference is in our endocrine system—our hormones. But have you ever seen a hormone?

Your Hormones Are the Boss

Despite being invisible, hormones influence everything in our bodies. They fundamentally determine our health, our vitality, and our moods. They determine if we build muscles and burn fat easily or if our fat stubbornly stays put no matter how much we devote ourselves to following a diet or going to the gym three times a week. Hormones control our fat stores. Our hormones determine whether we have cellulitis or not, how our hair, skin, and nails look, and whether we easily get stressed out or stay calm when times are tough. It's hormones that determine whether we wake up full of energy—or would kill someone for an extra hour's sleep.

Cravings aren't a sign that you lack willpower: they're your hormones sending you to the fridge. It's your hormones that make you engaged and content or anxious and depressed. It's your hormones that help you concentrate through a long meeting today and remember the important details from it tomorrow.

....

Cravings aren't a sign that you lack willpower:
they're your hormones sending you to the fridge.

....

**Your Hormones Determine Your Headaches, the Gloss
of Your Hair, Your Memory, and Your Happiness**

Few women make the connection between their host of symptoms and their hormones. Hot flashes, infertility, breast tenderness, irregular periods, and thyroid problems... we do link *these* symptoms to our hormones. But a healthy head of hair, a keen memory, a strong libido, robust energy, a good night's sleep, energy to go to the gym, and not needing to snack between meals? These are also symptoms of our hormones, albeit positive ones.

Magic results when your hormones are in balance: you feel energetic and cheerful; you're ready to spring into action; you have a good memory, you feel good, you glow, and you can experience deep contentment and gratitude, regardless of your age. Many women suffer from imbalanced hormones, but few understand hormone imbalance to be the cause of their symptoms. After all, where would we have learned this?

Society, including the medical world, focuses on fighting disease and chronic illness. But working on your health is a different process from fighting disease and illness while expecting others to solve these problems for you—and a much more fun one. I would rather focus on abundance and health, because everything that gets attention grows. The magic of health and vitality arises when we set our sights on health and vitality.

....

Working on our health and vitality is a
much more fun and powerful process than
fighting against disease and illness.

....

THE MAGIC OF HORMONES IN BALANCE

Do you experience too few of the "symptoms" below? You probably had them as a child. Would you gladly take them back, regardless of your age? These symptoms are all determined by your endocrine system:

- glowing skin
- healthy, thick hair
- strong nails
- a good mood, even during your period
- a slim waist
- the absence of headaches
- abundant energy
- knowing when you've eaten enough
- a stable, healthy weight without dieting
- a strong libido
- feeling happy and laughing often
- the courage and motivation to try new things

- curiosity
- the ability to relax, even during stressful times
- excellent sleep habits
- waking up with lots of energy
- motivation to move and exercise
- daily bowel movements
- mental sharpness and alertness
- a good memory
- eating regular meals without craving snacks
- feeling generally content for no particular reason
- crying only when the situation really warrants it
- having few wrinkles for your age
- having no hair growth where you shouldn't
- normal perspiration
- feet and hands that are neither hot nor cold
- good concentration
- a healthy metabolism

There is actually nothing in your body that is not influenced by your hormones. But it's only when all your hormones work in harmony with each other, when your endocrine system is in balance, that the magic occurs: you not only feel healthy, vital, and strong, but also feel confident, look great, and sleep well; your eyes shine, your emotions are in equilibrium, your mind is sharp, you experience deep joy, and you feel truly lucky and satisfied with yourself.

WOMEN ARE SENSITIVE TO HORMONE CHANGES

Almost nothing happens in your body that doesn't involve your hormones. Many "female complaints" are hormonal problems telling us that something is out of balance, because whether we like it or not, women are more sensitive to hormonal changes than men, and more vulnerable to hormone imbalance. Your hormones are constantly sending you messages to signal any imbalances. That's why it is wise to truly understand your hormones' influence: this will help you to grow old in good health.

....

When you get to know your hormones,
you'll have a powerful tool to help you
to a healthy and vital old age.

....

Quality of Life Starts with Balanced Hormones

If you think of hormones as being like the wiring system of a house, then men have a simple switch while women have a complex electrical panel. For men, testosterone plays the main role. This hormone starts to play an important role during puberty, quickly assumes the lead, and the switch is turned ON. After age 40, the switch slowly returns to the OFF position. This happens at a rate of approximately 2 percent change per year, and it's all fairly clear and predictable.

Women have a complex electrical panel because every month an egg is prepared in the uterus for fertilization. As a woman, you experience more hormonal swings in one month than a man does in a lifetime. Quality of life, and along with it the possibility of living up to your full potential, starts with hormones that are in balance with each other, that replace each other when necessary, that do what needs to be done to give you full energy and health.

You Have More Influence Than You Think

Do you sometimes feel like a victim of your hormones? Have you ever, in despair, called out "It's my hormones!" when you were being moody with your partner, only to ask yourself an hour later where that outburst came from? Do you sometimes have crying spells over nothing? Many women feel like they're victims of their hormones, but often they only mean by this their monthly hormone fluctuations—complaints such as premenstrual cravings or, later, menopause and its accompanying hot flashes. By now, though, I've shown you that the range of impact of your hormones is much larger than that. Your hormones are with you *every* day—you can't escape them.

....

Your hormones aren't adventurers doing their own thing.

....

I have good news for you: you no longer have to feel like a victim of your hormones. On the contrary—you have a lot of influence. And insight into hormonal housekeeping is an important tool to let you direct not only your health, vitality, and weight, but also your mental and emotional health. Yes, your mood too!

Your hormones aren't adventurers that do their own thing in your body and over which you have no say. If you know how they work, you can make them work *for* you instead of feeling like they're constantly working against you.

In fact, there's really no conflict, because you and your hormones want the same thing: to keep you healthy and happy as long as possible. Once you get to know your hormones and include them on your team, you'll have powerful supporters to keep you healthy and vital as long as possible. So how can you work together with your hormones?

Your Hormones Communicate with Your Environment

You can think of your hormones as bodyguards prepared to defend you 24-7. They continually scan the environment to gauge if it's safe for you. It might seem to you that your body is separate from your environment—after all, you can jump on a plane to Tahiti and remove your body from your current environment—but in reality your body is always responding to its surroundings. And that's a good thing because otherwise, you couldn't survive. When it's cold out in Montana, your body does its best to keep you warm, but if you deplane in tropical Tahiti, your body will do everything possible to help you cool off.

In fact your body is constantly communicating with its surroundings to determine what you need. Is it time to warm you up, or to cool you down? To go to sleep, or to wake up? To store fat, or to use your fat storage? Are you hungry right now or satiated? Would it make you happy to have sex at the moment, or would it be better to spend some time alone? Your body is never detached from its environment, and your hormones are constantly adapting to that environment to keep you healthy.

Your Environment Is Not Ideal for Your Hormones

Now we come to the core of the issue and the key to all hormonal problems: the circumstances your body finds itself in are not ideal. Your hormones would rather that you be outside all day in a wonderful climate, without any pollution, while you do nothing except wander around gathering vegetables, fruit, nuts, roots, and some insects, chat with other women, play with the children, and gather around the fire in the evening with your loved ones to prepare a delicious meal. Afterward, a wildly attractive man would invite you to dive into the bushes with him. I'm guessing that your reality is a little different than this. Mine is.

YOUR ENVIRONMENT IS MORE IMPORTANT THAN YOUR GENETICS

Ailments and diseases are often attributed to genetics. Your genes are not written in stone, though—in fact, they're as supple as a willow branch. Much research has been done with identical twins, who have the same genes and therefore exactly the same DNA. Turns out that they never lead exactly the same lives and seldom suffer from the same ailments or diseases. Indeed, their lives and their physical, mental, and emotional health can be quite different. Even with a high genetic disposition for certain diseases, one twin may be affected at age 33 and the other in her 80s—or even not at all. That's how powerful environmental influences are, and how weak genetics can be.

Women's Health Seems More Vulnerable

In Western society today, women's health seems more vulnerable than men's. Our average life span is 83, three and a half years longer than men, but we experience *seven* more years of assorted chronic diseases. Our extra years of life are of dubious quality. I don't like to be cynical, but from this statistic you could ask a bitter question: Do women live longer, or do we just die more slowly?

It's not only about the last seven years of our lives. As women, we experience a host of chronic diseases during our lifetime that men tend to avoid, and that's excluding the complaints that concern our female organs—our uteruses, ovaries, vaginas, and breasts.

In the Western world women are 15 times more likely to suffer the symptoms of an underactive thyroid. Rheumatoid arthritis, osteoarthritis, bone loss, chronic fatigue syndrome, Alzheimer's, brain aneurysms, cardiovascular diseases—all are more common in women. This is also true for autoimmune diseases such as Crohn's, Hashimoto's thyroiditis, celiac disease, and multiple sclerosis. Depression, anxiety, and insomnia afflict twice as many women as men. Female patients account for 75 percent of prescriptions for insomnia and depression—a billion-dollar industry. Furthermore, the number of women who suffer from poorly understood conditions such as PMS, polycystic ovary syndrome, endometrioses, painful menstruation, migraine, sore breasts, fibroids, hair loss, lipedema, thyroid problems, mood swings, adrenal gland issues, and memory loss is on the rise.

Poorly understood conditions are much more common in women than in men. One quarter of American women are medicated for mental health issues. Psychiatric departments are full of women, not men. More and more young women are experiencing fertility issues, and women suffer from diseases such as Alzheimer's and Parkinson's at younger ages. Many more women over 40 suffer from a broad scale of issues labeled as "menopause" or "perimenopause." One in three women will experience cancer. Breast cancer affects 1 in 8 women; in the 1950s, this number was just 1 in 22.

A worldwide epidemic continues to claim more victims. Never in human history have women been so unhealthy. What's going on? The answer is that we live in a world that increasingly disrupts the balance of our hormones. Men also experience hormonal disruptions, but women are more susceptible.

....
We live in a world that increasingly
disrupts our hormonal balance.
....

YOUR ENVIRONMENT DISRUPTS
YOUR HORMONE BALANCE

What are the most critical hormone disruptors threatening women's health?

DIET

Many critical disruptors of the endocrine system can be found in our diet. On the one hand, our diet is deficient in some essential factors, such as healthy fats, needed for a healthy female body. On the other hand, it's full of chemical additives that lead to hormonal chaos, the main culprits being xenoestrogens, a category of endocrine disruptors that have estrogen-like effects (*xeno* means "other" or "foreign"). Because xenoestrogens so closely resemble estrogen, women are much more sensitive to their impact than men. I'll return to this subject in detail in Chapter 2.

WEIGHT LOSS EFFORTS

We live in a world that puts a high value on being slim. For most women, this is an unhealthy mindset. Men are naturally more muscular; women naturally have some extra fat.

Have you ever pretzeled yourself to lose weight? You're not the only one. Women are much more likely than men to diet, with the result that they get fatter and less fit, because dieting completely disrupts the balance of women's endocrine systems. This leads to anguish and frustration and yet another diet as soon as the spring bulbs break ground. Diets wreak havoc on your hormones.

Yes, as a woman over the age of 40 you *can* become slim and maintain a healthy physique, but only if you're healthy first. It's often said that you need to lose weight to be healthy. But I prefer to turn this around: first you must be healthy, and then weight loss will happen naturally as a bonus. I'll explain how this works in Chapter 4.

THE QUEST FOR YOUTH AND BEAUTY

Being beautiful as long as possible is also highly valued by our society. And "beautiful" is synonymous with "looking young." We would prefer to avoid aging for as long as we can. Women in particular, it seems, must meet this expectation. How many different personal care products and cosmetics have you used today? To stay young-looking and beautiful, we women spend our lives smearing a cocktail of products on our skin, hair, and nails. Unbeknownst to us, many of these chemicals are endocrine disruptors absorbed by our bodies. Your skin absorbs up to 60 percent of the product you apply. Luckily, there are now excellent alternative products made of natural ingredients at a variety of price points. Do your hormones a favor and switch to a brand free of endocrine-disrupting and cancer-causing chemicals.

A COCKTAIL OF ENDOCRINE DISRUPTORS FOR YOUR SKIN?

Women use an average of 15 different cosmetics and personal care products per day. According to research by the Kyoto Prefectural University of Medicine, this means we're applying an average of 515 synthetic chemicals a day to our skin. Perfumes easily contain about 250. No researcher in the world is measuring the effects of these chemicals on our health.

TEN INGREDIENTS TO AVOID AT ALL COSTS

- parabens
- phthalates
- triclosan
- aluminum
- sodium lauryl (or sodium laureth) sulfate
- alcohol (also called ethanol)
- fragrance or parfum, a catchall for a variety of chemical substances
- butylated hydroxyanisole (BHA) or butylated hydroxytoluene (BHT)
- benzophenone-3 (oxybenzone)
- cocamidopropyl betaine

HOUSEHOLD PRODUCTS

Who does most of the housework in your home? These tasks still are largely the responsibility of women. Doing housework is another way to disrupt your endocrine system, because it also exposes you to many endocrine-disrupting chemicals. Cleaning products, laundry soap, dryer sheets, and herbicides for the weeds in your garden?

These products often contains chemicals that negatively affect your hormones.

MEDICATIONS

Please let me be clear, I am grateful for medication: it can save lives. But for most women long-term use of medication is not the solution for their problems. Many women spend years on contraceptive pills that suppress and disrupt the functioning of their hormones. Millions of women worldwide use the pill not for contraception but to mask myriad hormone dysfunctions, which inevitably are not solved. The longer a hormone problem exists, the more difficult it is to re-establish the balance of our endocrine system.

Have you taken medication for extended lengths of time? Medication may be necessary, but often it's not a remedy that actually heals. Only your body can heal itself. Even when surgeons and other specialists put your body back together after an accident, it's still your body that does the healing.

MOST MEDICATION HAS NEVER BEEN TESTED ON WOMEN

Until 1993 women (and female lab animaals) were systematically excluded from medical research. Scientists assumed that women's hormonal cycles or use of the pill would influence test results. But in everyday life women do have menstrual cycles and many women use the pill, so it's actually important to understand the influence of these things on the efficacy of medications! It is still the case that many established medications have never been studied for their effect on women. One study, the Knowledge Agenda on Gender and Health, commissioned by the Dutch Ministry of Health, Welfare, and Sport and published in 2015, showed that women have a 60 percent greater incidence of serious side effects from medications than do men.

The medical world has put little focus on the differences between men and women. Most doctors really do not understand how female hormones influence our lives. They have little knowledge about the female body and the complex ways in which hormones interact. There is still much clarity and understanding to be gained from further research. Doctors don't relate our complaints to our endocrine system, so many women are still sent home with the advice to "learn to live with it." Our doctors are fantastic when it comes to fixing something that's broken in our bodies but less good at helping us stay healthy.

··

It is never doctors that make you better;
it's ultimately your own body that does the healing.

··

That's why it's so important to become the manager of your own health. This is the time to learn more and to take responsibility. Knowledge and self-confidence are powerful medicine for women. Be aware that your doctor often doesn't have time for a thorough conversation with you—and the debilitating argument with your mother that caused your high blood pressure almost never comes up. There's a good chance that instead you'll be standing outside with a prescription for blood pressure medication. But high blood pressure isn't caused by a shortage of beta-blockers, just like a headache isn't due to a shortage of painkillers. There's always something else that's wrong.

Your doctor probably received no more than six hours of instruction on nutrition in their years of medical school. What doctor asks what you've got in your fridge and kitchen cupboards? You don't need a doctor to realize that nutrition and lifestyle have a huge influence on your health.

....

What doctor asks what you've got in your fridge and kitchen cupboards?

....

STRESS

I won't ask you because these days, what woman isn't stressed? Stress is bad for everyone. Stress is also the most powerful hormone disruptor. Although this is equally true for men, here too women draw the short straw because, thanks to our endocrine system, we're more sensitive to stress than men. Especially for women over 40, stress can really mess things up for you if you want to have a healthy body and a fantastic life. In Chapter 2 I'll explain how this works and why relaxation is critical for women over 40.

....

Stress is the most powerful hormone disruptor.

....

LACK OF PHYSICAL ACTIVITY

In an ideal environment, you'd be physically active most of the day. This is what makes your hormones happy. On average, we move only three hours a day, with the exception of weekends, when we're more active. By "move" I mean take part in activities such as walking, biking, housekeeping, and getting groceries. How many hours a day are you physically active? And do you also exercise? "Exercise" here can be anything that raises your heart rate and that you're doing to improve your skills and endurance. It could be cardio, circuit, interval, or weight training. Getting enough physical activity and exercise is important for your hormones.

Instead, are you seldom physically active, and do you rarely feel like exercising because you're too tired? An undernourished body has no desire to start moving. Start by improving your nutrition; the inspiration to be physically active will follow. Really—I promise you!

DO YOU WANT TO EARN MORE?
START WITH WEIGHT TRAINING!

As you age, your muscle strength slowly diminishes, unless you keep using your muscles fully. The older you get, the more important it is to exercise. The good news is that you can continue to build muscle to a very ripe old age. Fitness centers should actually be bursting with people over 40: they need weight training and challenging cardio workouts the most. It's up to you whether you'll be using a walker at age 80 or still hiking in the mountains—the choice is yours. A fun side effect discovered in an American study is that women get braver as they build muscle mass.[1] Women who took weight training felt less anxious about driving a car in a strange city and were prepared to ask their bosses for a raise. More muscles mean more testosterone, which results in more decisiveness and more guts. I can tell you from personal experience that this is true.

A DISRUPTED SLEEP CYCLE

Many women work as nurses and caregivers, as flight attendants, or in other shift work. Unfortunately, this is not conducive for your endocrine system. Your growth hormone is active only when you sleep, repairing your cells. The sleep hormone melatonin is a powerful antioxidant produced by your body to protect you from infection and the aging process. Even if you're not a shift worker, we've extended the day and shortened the night through artificial light, making it very likely that you suffer from sleep deprivation. Sleeping long and deeply is the healthiest thing you can do. Women are twice as likely to suffer from insomnia than men.

Do you see how chances are high that you live in an environment that's not conducive to a balanced endocrine system? That is why it's so important to know what your hormones need if you're to function as optimally as possible.

WORK WITH YOUR HORMONES

If you want to build a super smart team with your hormones, it's important to realize that your hormones are always as busy as they're able to be keeping you healthy. Your job is to give the body full of those hormones the most beneficial environment possible. That's why it's important to learn about your hormones, because collaboration is much smarter than fighting. More critically, fighting your hormones is futile—it's a battle you'll always lose. Your hormones are many times stronger than your willpower. Does this frustration sound familiar? You've vowed to stop snacking, but you succumb to a piece of chocolate. Or this one: you intend to go to the gym twice a week but after three weeks you're already trying to find excuses not to go. These are examples of your willpower fighting against your hormones. How often have you experienced this?

But it's not hard for you to work together with your hormones, because your body functions logically. Let me give you an example.

Your Survival Instinct Will
Always Defeat Your Willpower

If you're watching TV late at night, you're telling your body it's still daytime. Your hormones don't understand TVs or computers, only day and night. Many women experience cravings late at night. Does that sound like you? Maybe this has caused you years of frustration, but for your hormones it's logical. Even at 11 o'clock at night, if you're sitting in artificial light, you're signaling to your hormones that it's broad daylight, and at the same time your hormones feel you getting tired. For your body, being tired in broad daylight signals danger, because your attention may drift. Your hormones don't know that you're lazily watching a movie on the couch or sitting at your computer with danger nowhere to be seen.

But imagine if you suddenly had to run from a bear or, as might be more likely in our reality, put out a fire started by candles that were left too close to the curtains. How are you best prepared to respond? By making sure there's some energy in reserve. How do you get that energy? By eating—preferably something that gives you energy quickly. For your hormones, this is totally logical. So even if you've vowed not to snack tonight, your survival instinct will always defeat your willpower. And that's how those last six cookies in the jar or those last slices of pizza disappear...

Now do you understand why it's important to understand how your hormones "think"? If you know how they work, it's not as hard to, in this example of late-night snacking, give your body the signal that it's late and that you're safe. An hour before bedtime, turn off the TV and computer, dim the lights, listen to relaxing music, and take a book to bed or run yourself a bath. If you're tired, go to bed on time and avoid the temptation to quickly dive back into the online universe. You'll notice that your hormones will crave sweets and other snacks way less often.

THE MOST IMPORTANT ENVIRONMENT MAY BE YOUR DIET

Your hormones react directly to your environment. But putting yourself in a healthier environment does not, fortunately, mean as radical a change as emigrating to sunny Tahiti. The most important type of environment may be your diet: it's the environment you invite into your body.

You are what you eat, at a far deeper level than you probably realize. Every second 10 million cells die in your body, and 10 million new ones are produced. They achieve this because of what you feed yourself. Your body is a structure that constantly rebuilds and heals itself. A cut on your finger and a bruise on your leg heal themselves. This healing process also happens deep inside, where you can't see it.

Every Second Millions of New Cells Are Produced Because of Your Diet

We're talking about massive cell renewal thanks to what you eat. Not only your hair and nails but also your heart, your liver, your kidneys, and even your bones consist of living tissue that is constantly renewing and repairing itself. Your diet determines whether your body has enough nutrients to rebuild itself every second with healthy cells. Your diet also determines if you have enough nutrients to produce the right hormones in the right amount.

Tomorrow's Body Is Lying on Your Plate Today

What you eat is important. I like to say, "Tomorrow's body is lying on your plate today." Actually, that's too simplistic, because it's also important that your body can absorb these nutrients, use them appropriately, and dispose of them appropriately. In the worst-case scenario, you eat valuable nutrients but poop them back out unused. The healthier you eat, the more your body and digestive system will rebalance themselves and the better you'll digest and absorb valuable nutrients.

Diet has an enormous influence on your brain and emotions too. There's a direct relationship between what you eat and your ability to concentrate, and also your mental health and emotional state. Your diet has enormous influence on your hormones, and your hormones largely determine how you feel. In Chapter 2, I'll go into greater detail.

Some cells in your body replace themselves in a day and others take longer, but within seven years pretty much every cell in your body has been replaced. This means that in seven years you can be a totally new person! How you'll look and feel then is largely determined by what you put on your plate every day.

The Food on Your Plate: A Starting Point for Change

In my experience, and for many of the women I guide, the food on your plate is a critical starting point for change. If you begin to feed yourself properly, your hormones will mostly rebalance themselves. Food cravings will disappear because a well-nourished body is not begging for nutrients. You'll also notice that you sleep better, and as a result have more energy. More sleep means you're more relaxed too. You'll notice that it will be easier to achieve a healthy weight. Hopefully, you'll never go on another weight-loss diet, which will help you avoid a significant endocrine disruptor. A healthy diet will also give you more energy to be active so you'll make fewer excuses to avoid the gym. Really—a healthy body *wants* to be active! Good nutrition will make you feel healthier, and that will make you look better, which will improve your self-esteem. Maybe you'll finally decide to look for a better job, or it will be easier for you to say "no" without feeling guilty, and that will afford you more time to do the things that are important to you.

The Nutrition Compass is my advice for all women who want to rebalance their endocrine system. This is the beginning of the journey to more vitality and health. A healthy body can enable you to create the life you want, whether you're young or already past menopause. But first let me tell you a few more things about menopause, because there are a lot of misunderstandings out there.

MENOPAUSE IS NEVER THE PROBLEM

The biggest myth is that your health automatically declines after the age of 40. If you constantly tell yourself that your health will decline after 40, then this will become your truth: your body is influenced by what you think. Thoughts are even more powerful than hormones. That's why your convictions about aging are important if you want to age with health and vitality.

There's another conviction you can choose: you can live to a ripe old age full of health and vitality—physically, mentally, and emotionally. In the last few years this has become my conviction. This is the narrative that I would love you to believe in too.

My goal with this book is to help you work together with your endocrine system so that you can get to at least 85 full of health and vitality. And that's why I can't avoid talking about menopause, a time when many women experience all sorts of health complaints that are attributed to our hormones.

....

Let's not blame women's bodies for
our menopause symptoms.

....

Menopause Lasts Only a Day

Lots has been written about menopause and perimenopause, the time leading up to menopause. Books, and the internet, contain a tsunami of complaints associated with this time in our lives—as if menopause were to blame for all of them. If we're not careful, we're going to start believing that too.

The symptoms associated with menopause can begin around age 45 (often earlier) and can last about 10 years. They usually occur years before our last menstruation, which happens when we're around 52. After that the symptoms often diminish, but not for everyone, because each woman is unique. *Menopause* is the word for one day one whole year after your last period. You only know it was your last period once you haven't menstruated for one year. After that you no longer need to use birth control, although I know a host of healthy women over the age of 50 who don't trust that guarantee. So in fact menopause lasts for only a day. That's good news, isn't it?

However, we tend to attribute just about any health issue between the ages of 45 and 55 to menopause. It can end up seeming as if everything that changes in our bodies during that time is part of menopause.

When we blame all our problems for a decade on menopause, it suggests that Nature made a mistake in creating women's bodies. I'm convinced this is simply not true. That is why I like to say: menopause lasts for only one day.

Please note, I'm the last person to trivialize the challenges of perimenopause and menopause, because I know they're real, both physically and mentally. I've experienced my own share of them. Especially if you're under a lot of stress between 45 and 55, your endocrine system will be wildly out of balance and you'll experience many symptoms. But it's really not our (peri)menopause that's to blame for these annoying and severe symptoms. Once again it's the environment we live in, the things around us that disrupt our sensitive hormones and cause these issues.

Perimenopause Symptoms Are Largely Determined by Where You Live

In Western society, 80 percent of women experience hot flashes, and it can make their lives very difficult. As women in the developing world adopt Western lifestyle and nutrition habits, they too develop these symptoms. At the same time, many Western women sail through menopause symptom-free. The logical conclusion is that it's not so much the female body itself that is to blame as it is the environment and circumstances in which we find ourselves. Most symptoms associated with menopause (including weight gain) and many chronic diseases in the Western world are the result of our lifestyle, dietary habits, and environment. The time leading up to menopause is one when women are extra-sensitive to hormonal upheaval. That's why so many symptoms are more obvious then. Until you're 40, your body looks after you. After that, you and your body must work together wisely. So at 40 it's time to take action!

It's Never Too Soon to Start Dealing with Menopause

I cannot emphasize enough that your body functions intelligently and amazingly. If you work with your hormones, menopause will not be a time full of complaints and discomfort. Instead it will be a time of transformation and growth and blossoming.

When your body sends you signals in the form of complaints and illness, look at these as requests for help. Usually these requests begin as whispers, but if you don't listen to the soft whispers and ignore the minor issues, your body will call louder, and eventually it will light an emergency flare. If your body is sending you cries for help after you turn 45, it usually means you've ignored the whispers for years. Women are very good at that: we ignore the signals of minor pain and discomfort until our bodies start using heavier artillery.

Hormonal imbalance often exists long before the lead-up to menopause begins. Sometimes I ask, "Is your body leaving you in the lurch, or is it the other way around?"

Menopause Complaints:
The Last Wake-up Call

Aches and pains and minor complaints are wake-up calls to listen to your body and take steps to form a smart team. Pay attention to the minor signals: they can be as simple as a bit of pain, a spot of eczema that won't go away, or a recurring cold sore. If at 45 you no longer feel bubbly and energetic, how will you feel at 55? Or 85? Between 45 and 55 we begin to experience symptoms we conveniently call menopause problems. The ten most common are:

- hot flashes and night sweats
- vaginal dryness
- weight gain
- sleep problems
- exhaustion
- headaches
- low libido
- mood swings
- depressive episodes or depression
- heavy periods

If you look closely, you'll note that these symptoms are not experienced only by women 45 and older. The exceptions might be hot flashes, night sweats, and vaginal dryness—the menopause-specific symptoms. The others on the list can also be experienced by younger women and by men.

ARE MENOPAUSE SYMPTOMS RESTRICTED TO WOMEN?

In their book *Check Your Best Before Date*, Pim Christiaans and Hanny Roskamp write that the best-kept secret of endocrinologists is that older men experience the same symptoms as women, from hot flashes to mood swings. And we all know what Viagra is for. So maybe even those female-specific menopause symptoms—hot flashes, night sweats, and sexual arousal problems—are not so typically feminine.

Menopause symptoms are the sum of everything that happened before. Because of hormonal changes, a woman's body is more vulnerable during this time, which is why these symptoms become more prominent. Menopause is the last wake-up call on the path to aging full of health and vitality.

In other words, it's never too soon to start dealing with menopause. If you begin to work with your hormones early enough, there's a good chance that the road to menopause will give you very few physical and emotional problems, that it will energize you instead!

In the next chapter, I'll introduce you to your most important hormones and organs so that you can discover if you're already a good team or if there is room for improvement.

REMEMBER THIS

· In many ways, your hormones determine your health, vitality, and appearance.

- Your hormones want you to live a long and happy life.
- Your endocrine system becomes imbalanced in the environment of an unhealthy diet, too much stress, too little exercise, not enough sleep, and too many toxic chemicals.
- Once you understand how your hormonal system works, it will be easier to work together and become a super smart team.
- Nutrition is an important starting point for changing your life. Change your diet, change your hormones, change your life.
- Menopause is often associated with a long list of symptoms. Whether you experience these symptoms depends in large part on your environment.

GREEN SMOOTHIE

I find smoothies the ideal way to get some green vegetables at the start of the day. Make sure your smoothie has enough fat and protein, or you'll be hungry again an hour later. On top of that, fats promote the absorption of vitamins and minerals in your intestines. Here's one of my favorite recipes, one with endless possible variations. I love to eat this with a spoon out of a wide bowl.

Here's What You Need
1 tablespoon rolled oats
1 orange
a handful of spinach (about ¼ cup)
half a ripe banana
1 kiwi
7 tablespoons nondairy milk
1 tablespoon shelled hemp seeds

Here's How You Make It
Soak the rolled oats overnight in a bit of water. With a sharp knife, peel the orange as you would an apple, and quarter. This way, you also get the seeds and roughage, and all the nutrients.

Put all the ingredients in a blender and blend to a thick paste. Taste to see what else it needs. Sometimes I add a squirt of lemon juice. Pour the mixture into a wide bowl. Sprinkle liberally with hempseed for extra protein. Feel free to top with grated coconut, chopped nuts or seeds, or the rest of the thinly sliced banana.

2

WORK WISELY WITH YOUR HORMONES

UNDERSTANDING MY HORMONES and how I could influence them positively was the most important key to my recovery from burnout. It also gave me a boost in energy and well-being that has lasted to this day. I now know that as a woman I need a deep understanding of my endocrine system. I just wish I'd learned this earlier in my life.

....

Rebalancing your hormones is much easier than living with hormonal chaos in your body.

....

YOUR HORMONES ARE THE INSTRUMENTS IN YOUR ORCHESTRA

In this chapter, I'll introduce you to the seven most important hormones and two key organs. While I'll describe them individually, they work together so closely that you can't regard them as separate. They work together like musicians in an orchestra. Every orchestra member is unique, has their own instrument and role. Beautiful music is created when all the members play at their best and work together appropriately.

I thought long and hard about whether to give you tips about individual hormones, tips you could begin to use immediately. I didn't want to because you shouldn't consider your hormones as separate from one another. It's better to understand them all together. The Nutrition Compass is my complete method for you to rebalance your hormones by using nutrition. But after skimming the headings in this chapter, I can imagine that you can't wait to get to work, so I decided to break it down for the sake of accessibility.

Trying Counts

Keep in mind that each body is unique. Something that delivers great results for one woman may not work for another. It's always a matter of discovering what works for *you*. Be curious. Try different things. When it comes to your health, effort is what matters. Additionally, realize that your body is slow to change as an organism. Adding flaxseed to your diet today doesn't mean you'll feel the results or see them in the mirror the day after tomorrow.

YOU ARE UNIQUE; SO IS YOUR HORMONE BALANCE

After reading many complicated studies and thick books written by doctors about the female hormones, I can tell you that specialists in women's health and scientists often disagree. With their "measuring is knowing," "prove it," and mechanical view of the body, they still have not successfully fathomed the mystery of the female body. There is still so much we do not understand, because every woman's body is unique.

This is not to say we know nothing—scientists do agree on the broad strokes. Luckily, that's enough, because your body understands the details when it comes to achieving a balanced endocrine system. For your body, balancing your endocrine system is a task no more difficult than keeping your heart beating, keeping your digestive system working, and making sure you continue to breathe while you sleep. It's only when your environment has disrupted this balance that your body needs your help. Unfortunately, in our society this is often the case.

What Are Hormones?

Your hormones are chemicals that are produced in various parts of your body. You can imagine them as important messengers transported (mainly) through your bloodstream to all sorts of cells, with instructions about what the cells need to do. Once the hormones' work is done, they're broken down in the liver and intestines and then eliminated. Your body creates hundreds of different hormones, but a few are critical, and it would be wise to get to know them.

Hormone Balance Is Always in Flux

Many people think of balance working like a scale or seesaw, but hormone balance is more complex than that. It looks more like this:

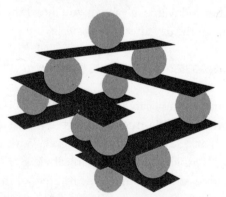

Don't get discouraged, though—it isn't as complicated as it looks. Your body intrinsically knows how to achieve this balance, because it's uniquely equipped for that task. Let's just say that the important part for you is to provide the essential building blocks and ensure that a hard wind doesn't blow the whole structure down.

Your body continually strives to maintain balance. It is constantly monitoring stimuli that threaten that balance and constantly working hard to counteract them. When danger threatens, your hormones give you a shot of extra energy so you can run away fast; if you're too hot, your body will sweat to help cool you off; when you notice a bad smell, it warns you to be careful and determine the cause (did you leave the propane tank on?); when you smell a freshly baked apple pie, you'll crave a piece. These are all healthy "imbalances." Your body reacts to them and then rebalances itself. I prefer to use the term *dynamic hormone equilibrium.*

DYNAMIC HORMONE EQUILIBRIUM

Each month during your fertile years, your body will try to ripen an egg, or oocyte. Your pituitary gland—a small organ in your brain—creates FSH, follicle-stimulating hormone, for this process. FSH ensures that the follicle, a fluid-filled sac that encases an oocyte in your ovaries, helps the oocyte mature. The hormone estrogen is produced due to the maturation of the egg in its follicle. Estrogen, among other things, helps to build the mucous membrane in your uterus so that the fertilized egg can be nourished. After about 14 days, the estrogen tells your pituitary gland that your uterus is ready, upon which your pituitary gland produces a big surge of LH, luteinizing hormone, which triggers the ovulation.

During ovulation, the mature egg is released from the follicle, ready to meet and be fertilized by a sperm cell. The empty follicle then produces the hormone progesterone, which has multiple jobs, including managing the implantation of the fertilized egg. Progesterone now takes the lead role, and the production of estrogen decreases. If the egg doesn't encounter a nice sperm cell, the uterus lining is expelled with the egg, and the cycle begins again.

(Did you know that the egg chooses the sperm cell? It's not at all true that the first sperm it encounters will win!) Do you see how dynamic, yet vulnerable, this dance of the female hormones is? There's so much involved!

BASIC RULES FOR DYNAMIC HORMONE EQUILIBRIUM

The most important thing to know is that too much or too little of certain active hormones in your body for too long is not healthy. That is the main rule. Your body maintains a healthy, dynamic balance of enough active hormones on the one hand and the excretion of spent hormones on the other. It's only when there are too many active hormones or not enough that things start to go wrong.

Enough Production: Of Active Hormones

"Enough" when it comes to hormone production means not too much and not too little. If an organ does produce too much of a certain hormone, your body has a host of methods to remedy this:

· It can increase the excretion of this hormone.
· It can convert the hormone into a different hormone.
· It can temporarily inactivate a certain amount of those hormones.
· It can make your cells unresponsive to that hormone in order to minimize the potential damage it could cause.

Insulin, for example, is a hormone that gets to work when your blood contains glucose (sugar) that needs to be delivered to your cells. Insulin ensures that the cells can absorb the glucose. If insulin is constantly working in overdrive, your cells will eventually become less sensitive to it, which means that they'll stop absorbing glucose. We call this being "insulin resistant," and it can be the beginning of an avalanche of problems. Luckily, the problem can be reversed and your cells can once again become receptive to insulin.

If your body is producing too little of a certain hormone, that hormone can sometimes be replaced by another. This is how progesterone can be converted into estrogen but also into cortisol if your body needs cortisol more.

Hormone-producing organs can also take over each other's production of several hormones. After the age of 30, your ovaries slowly but surely produce less estrogen and progesterone. Because your body still needs to produce sufficient estrogen later in life, the task is slowly transferred to your adrenal glands, your skin, your muscles, and your fat cells. When production of one type of hormone decreases, this is how your body ensures hormonal balance.

Sufficient Elimination: Of Spent Hormones

Balance is not just about adequate production: the appropriate breakdown and elimination of spent hormones is at least as important. Things often go wrong at this stage, and too much of one kind of hormone remains in your body. Your body tries everything to dispose of spent hormones. If it can't manage the elimination, the hormones are temporarily stored in the place in your body that will cause the least harm.

**Adequate Storage: Your Fat Cells Are the
Safest Storage Place for Estrogen**

Overproduction of estrogen can cause serious health issues. To avoid this damage, your body stores it in a safe place: your fat cells. The more surplus estrogen, the more storage required. Existing fat cells may swell, but with a surplus of estrogen your body may also decide to create new fat cells.[1] This is stubborn fat—hard to get rid of. It's up to you to make it easier for your body to dispose of surplus estrogen. Be sure to read further if you want to learn how to do this.

....
Your hormones are like bowling pins:
if one gets knocked over, it
usually takes a couple more with it.
....

THE MOST IMPORTANT TEAM MEMBERS

That brings us to your team. Let me introduce you to your most important hormones:
- the duo of estrogen and progesterone
- insulin
- cortisol
- thyroid hormones
- the duo of leptin and ghrelin

It's also important to become acquainted with the two most important organs when it comes to dynamic hormone balance: your intestines and your liver. Together they are responsible for the sufficient production and expulsion of hormones.

One Hormone Out of Balance? So Are Others

Your hormones work together ingeniously. On the one hand, this is great, but the fact that hormones are tied so closely together has its drawbacks when it boomerangs back on us: if one is out of balance, there are always others out of balance too.

It therefore doesn't make much sense to talk about only one hormone. Cause and effect are often difficult to distinguish, and the same symptoms can result from a variety of hormonal imbalances. I once visited a group of women in a developing country. They were doing laundry in a river. They stood with their feet in the flowing water and spread out the clothes on round boulders as they applied soap. When I tried to explain how a washing machine worked, one of the women asked, "But how does a machine know where the stains are?"

Put Your Whole Body in the Wash

Your body works holistically: everything works together. You will achieve better health and more vitality only if you put your *whole* body into the "washing machine" instead of just scrubbing at a stain here and there. Your body isn't like a car, where you don't have to worry about the oil level when you have a flat tire. Your body is much more complex than that. One off-balance hormone can drag a bunch of others down with it, creating a vicious cycle.

THE VICIOUS CYCLE OF HORMONE IMBALANCE

If too much insulin is circulating in your blood, you can end up with a shortage of the sleep hormone melatonin and will sleep badly. Too little melatonin means too little cortisol in the morning, so you wake up tired. Melatonin also affects your satiety hormone, leptin, which then no longer works. With too little cortisol *and* too little leptin, chances are you'll crave sources of fast energy, such as sweets, all day long. Eating too many sweets results in too much insulin in your blood. If there's too much insulin circulating in your blood, you can end up with a shortage of the sleep hormone melatonin... and so on and so on.

The Points of the Nutrition Compass
Are Your Washing Machine

To get you started quickly on the road to health, I've provided some basic tips for each hormone. But remember: if you want to get your "laundry" really clean, you should put it *all* in the machine. Getting rid of stains here and there will not give you great results. Together, the seven points of the Nutrition Compass are the full wash cycle.

....

Try to understand how your hormones interact
and work together. Only then can you know
what's wrong and how you can best intervene.

....

REMEMBER THIS

· Your hormones are like messengers in your body, constantly telling all your cells what to do.
· Keeping your hormones in a good dynamic balance is normal
  everyday work for your body. Your body has many options at its
  disposal for restoring hormonal disbalance by itself.
· Too much or too little of any one hormone for too long a time is
  not healthy and will lead to problems.
· If your body can't manage to stay in balance any longer, then it's
  up to you to change the environment.

THE ENERGETIC WOMAN'S GRANOLA

This is my delicious Energetic Woman's Granola, full of healthy nutrients. Oats are an extraordinary grain that, in contrast to other grains, provide a *slow* rise in your blood sugar levels. They contain a lot of tryptophan, a component of serotonin, the happiness hormone. Cinnamon helps keep your blood sugar level stable. You can add chopped dried fruit, but you'll find the granola is already naturally quite sweet.

Here's What You Need

1⅔ cups rolled oats
⅓ cup sunflower seeds
⅓ cup pumpkin seeds
⅓ cup walnuts, finely chopped
⅓ cup cashews
⅓ cup dried coconut

½ teaspoon Ceylon cinnamon
½ teaspoon pure vanilla powder
zest of 1 organic lemon
3 tablespoons plus 1 teaspoon
    agave syrup

Here's How You Make It

Preheat the oven to 250°F.

Mix the rolled oats, seeds, nuts, and dried coconut in a large bowl. In a small bowl, mix together the cinnamon, vanilla, lemon zest, and agave syrup. Pour the agave mixture into the oat mixture and mix thoroughly.

Cover a baking sheet with ungreased parchment paper. Spread the mixture evenly over the baking sheet. Bake the granola in the oven for 45 minutes or until it is completely dry. If you have a small baking sheet, you may have to stir the mixture from time to time with a wooden spoon. Turn the oven off and leave the sheet of granola in it to cool. Store this delicious granola in an airtight container.

1. ESTROGEN AND PROGESTERONE: A DELICATE DANCE

Estrogen and progesterone are essential hormones that dance together: sometimes there's more estrogen, sometimes more progesterone, and that's exactly as it should be. These two hormones have leading roles in everything related to fertility and pregnancy, but it's just as important to keep them in balance after your fertile years.

Estrogen is the hormone that is mainly produced by your ovaries for most of your life. To be precise, there are three different kinds of estrogen: estrone, estradiol, and estriol, of which estradiol is the most important. Estrone is produced in fatty tissue, including your breasts, and will increase, relatively speaking, after menopause.

One of estrogen's many tasks is mitosis, or cell division: under its influence you develop breasts and rounder hips during puberty. About five years before menopause, your ovaries' estrogen production will begin to diminish. For the rest of your life this task will be taken over, in lesser amounts, by your adrenal glands, your skin, your muscles, and your fat cells. Your body continues to produce estrogen in your older years even though your ovaries are no longer responsible for this task, and that is a very good thing.

....

> A large portion of female complaints are caused by a disturbance in the balance between estrogen and progesterone.

....

ESTROGEN IS A MULTITASKER

Estrogen has over 400 essential functions in your body, including influencing your fertility, energy levels, joints, mucous membranes, libido, and skin quality. Estrogen is also responsible for delivering oxygen and glucose to your brain, regulating many mental functions.

It has a huge influence on your mood, memory, and ability to concentrate. It's no wonder your body ensures that you have some estrogen production till a ripe old age—you still need it. Remember the most basic rule of balanced hormones: too much or too little of any one hormone is not good for you. So when is there typically too much or not enough estrogen?

LOW-ESTROGEN DEPRESSION

Low estrogen levels lead to less production of serotonin. A shortage of serotonin doesn't feel good: it can flood you with depressive feelings, unexplained anxiety, lack of sexual desire, and abrupt, unexplained mood swings that make you feel like you're going crazy. You are not crazy: your body is just not producing enough estrogen, and thus not enough serotonin. During these moments, it is almost impossible to resist cravings, because sweets and carbohydrates temporarily raise your dopamine levels, which creates feelings of joy and contentment.

Dopamine and serotonin are chemicals— neurotransmitters—produced by your body to give you feelings of happiness and contentment.

INSUFFICIENT ESTROGEN, MOSTLY AFTER MENOPAUSE

When is there typically not enough estrogen? Low estrogen levels can occur
- temporarily, during the second half of your menstrual cycle, or
- long-term, leading up to or after menopause.

About five years before the onset of menopause, your ovaries reduce their production of estrogen. This might coincide with a lot of fluctuations, peaks and valleys in your cycle. You may suffer from these fluctuations; some women are more sensitive to them than others. Low estrogen levels are often blamed for hot flashes, exhaustion, and mood swings.

Low estrogen levels also influence two other chemicals: dopamine and serotonin. These chemicals produce feelings of happiness and contentment. Your body needs enough estrogen to produce these chemicals.

Uncontrollable Premenstrual Food Cravings

Temporary low estrogen levels relative to progesterone levels can make you extremely hungry. Many women notice this during the two weeks between ovulation and menstruation. It explains the cravings just before your period starts: your body points you to the box of chocolates in the back of the cupboard, and your willpower is no match for it.

Dopamine is also produced by your body when you use opium, nicotine, or marijuana, which are therefore all addictive. It's no wonder many women claim to be addicted to sweets, bread, potatoes, pizza, ice cream, or chocolate during the second half of their monthly cycle. Chocolate is many women's favorite, possibly because it contains magnesium, a nutrient many women commonly lack, plus a chemical called phenylethylamine, which plays a role in the production of serotonin.

The minute your period starts, the cravings stop. Consider yourself lucky if these cravings last only a couple of days, because many women suffer from them two weeks out of every four.

You can influence your estrogen levels through your diet. Hunger and extreme cravings during the second half of your cycle are usually the result of fluctuating blood sugar levels combined with insulin resistance. That is why you should follow my tips to avoid too much insulin or insulin resistance (page 74) and try to keep your blood sugar levels as stable as possible, especially during the first two weeks of your cycle. Following the points in the Nutrition Compass will also help reduce food cravings.

....

Stable blood sugar levels
will help you achieve a balance of
estrogen and progesterone.

....

Long-Term Shortage of Estrogen and Menopause

The estrogen levels in your body decline slowly but surely leading up to and during menopause. This is as nature intended, but the fluctuations in estrogen, especially relative to progesterone, can result in problems. Typical symptoms of low estrogen include:

- hot flashes and night sweats
- foggy memory and concentration problems
- prolonged fatigue
- mood swings
- signs of depression
- sleep problems
- low libido
- painful joints
- loss of bone density
- dry mucous membranes (eyes, vagina)
- dry skin and hair
- heart palpitations, dizziness
- feeling hungry

Sooner or later many women will experience some or most of these symptoms. Some women are more sensitive than others to the slow decline of their estrogen levels and to the fluctuations of estrogen relative to progesterone. I'll come back to this in the next section.

Estrogen Helps Prevent Wrinkles

Maybe you've noticed that many slim women around the age of 60 have more wrinkles. This is mostly because they have few fat cells and can therefore manufacture only a small amount of estrogen. Your body needs a certain amount of estrogen both to function well and to keep wrinkles at bay. This may well be why many women gain a few pounds during menopause. The body can produce extra estrogen thanks to these fat cells.

....

Body fat is hormonally active tissue: it can produce estrogen and testosterone.

....

When I explained this to a client who complained she'd always been slim but had suddenly developed a spare tire around the age of 55, she said, "So I have to choose between wrinkles and a spare tire?" I told her there was a third option: strength training. Strength training builds muscle, and muscle in turn produces testosterone. Thanks to the enzyme aromatase, this testosterone can be converted to estrogen. Strength training has many benefits for women.

You might be wondering why many women who are already overweight still gain a bit of weight during menopause. Maybe you can relate to this? There can be many reasons for it. In Chapter 4 I'll revisit this topic.

HOT FLASHES CAN RUIN YOUR LIFE

In 1967 we landed on the moon, but we still don't know exactly what a hot flash is. It has something to do with a disruption in the signal between your brain and your body as a result of hormonal fluctuations. Unfortunately, no one solution works for all women.

Hot flashes are aggravated by anything that causes stress, so avoid sugars, dairy, gluten, refined foods, coffee, alcohol, smoking, and external sources of stress. Make sure you get enough physical activity and rest. Drink enough water and eat healthy fats: there's a link between eating too few healthy fats and hot flashes. Maca root can help, as can herbs such as monk's pepper (vitex, or chasteberry) and black cohosh root. Some women benefit from acupuncture and respiratory therapy. If none of this provides any relief and you find your daily life compromised by hot flashes, seek the advice of a doctor or endocrinologist regarding appropriate hormone therapy.

TIPS FOR LOW ESTROGEN

EAT FRESHLY GROUND FLAXSEED.

Flax seeds contain lignans, which are phytoestrogens (plant-derived estrogens that resemble the body's estrogen). If your body is short on estrogen, these phytoestrogens can help balance estrogen levels. Grind the flax seeds in a blender or electric coffee grinder. Ground flax spoils quickly; store it in small portions, in a sealed glass jar, in your fridge. Flaxseed oil does not contain lignans.

ADD MACA TO YOUR SMOOTHIE.

The superfood maca is an adaptogen that stimulates the endocrine system to rebalance itself. The effects of maca on the female endocrine system have been documented.[2]

AVOID GLUTEN AND DAIRY AS MUCH AS POSSIBLE.

For the reliable function of your endocrine system, including the influence of estrogen on your dopamine and serotonin levels, you need healthy intestines—90 percent of serotonin is produced in healthy intestines. Gluten and dairy can disrupt healthy intestinal function.

TAKE A REGULAR MAGNESIUM BATH.

Many women suffer from a shortage of magnesium. Research has shown that the mineral magnesium can help alleviate the symptoms of low estrogen levels. Magnesium also helps with relaxation. Regularly add magnesium (Epsom salts) to your bath or footbath.

ENJOY RAW CACAO.

Raw cacao is a powerful source of magnesium.

EXCESS ESTROGEN, MOSTLY FROM EXTERNAL DISRUPTORS

It is much more common for the female body to have an elevated estradiol-to-progesterone ratio than the opposite. This is called *estrogen dominance* and means that there is a serious disruption in your endocrine system. It has been said that 80 percent of women in the Western world suffer from estrogen dominance.

Estrogen Dominance

In cases of estrogen dominance, it is often assumed that the body is producing too much estrogen. That can happen, especially in cases of obesity, because the fat cells can produce extra estrogen. However, the main cause of estrogen dominance is not the body itself but chemicals in our environment that resemble estrogen. Once they enter your body, these chemicals behave just like estrogen. They're called *xenoestrogens*.

Xenoestrogens have the same effect in our bodies as estrogens, but they are far stronger. These chemicals are commonly derived from the petrochemical industry—they're found in crude oil.

FROM CRUDE OIL TO
THOUSANDS OF PRODUCTS

You probably don't consider crude oil a natural product, but it is. Crude oil originates as the pressed remains of plants and animals that are millions of years old. Toward the end of the 1800s, the chemical industry realized it could make all kinds of products from crude oil. The processing of crude oil resulted in plastics, medications, fabrics, herbicides, cleaning products, pesticides, gasoline, dyes, sweeteners, and flavor enhancers, just to name a few. Crude oil can be found in small amounts in almost all processed foods. It is also found in meat and milk products, because animals eat feed that has been treated with pesticides and also routinely receive antibiotics. It can be found in products such as soap, shampoo, nail polish, cosmetics, personal care products, and perfumes. You can encounter it in carpets, furniture, paint, and building materials. Over 100,000 chemicals are in use, and every year another 1,000 or so are added. Despite all the processing, your female body still recognizes the natural origin—the crude oil—so it still has an effect on your body.

....
The main cause of estrogen dominance is not the body's own estrogen, but xenoestrogens.
....

I often talk about a "tsunami of xenoestrogens," because we cannot escape them. Running away won't help. Handling them intelligently will, and it's necessary, because having too much estrogen in your body results in a slow poisoning.

....

Estrogen dominance can result in a legion of problems in your body.

....

THE MOST COMMON ISSUES CAUSED
BY ESTROGEN DOMINANCE

The most common complaints caused by estrogen dominance—complaints that can worsen as the situations drags on—are fatigue; fluid retention and swelling; increased fat storage in the legs, hips, and breasts; stubborn obesity; cellulitis; low libido; heavy and/or painful periods; insomnia; night sweats; mood swings; polycystic ovary syndrome (PCOS); premenstrual syndrome (PMS); fibromyalgia; hormonal migraine; anxiety attacks; depression; hair loss; gallbladder issues; thyroid issues; endometriosis; painful breasts; breast cysts; fibroids; and all hormone-sensitive forms of cancer. See how these are symptoms and illnesses that occur much more often in women than in men?

WOMEN ARE MORE VULNERABLE

A woman's endocrine system is more vulnerable to all those xeno-estrogens than a man's is. That has something to do with the fact that the balance between estrogen and progesterone is more important in women than in men.

Too much estrogen in humans and other animals has an impact on their fertility; we sometimes hear this described as an "overdose" of the female hormone estrogen. Scientists around the world are seeing the results of this contamination—polar bears with both male and female sex organs, male frogs that develop ovaries, and male fish and turtles with female sex organs.[3] Everything in nature is becoming confused by this overdose of female hormones.

MEN ARE NOT IMMUNE

One in seven men in the Western world has a fertility problem. The decrease in sperm quality and the increase in prostate cancer are associated with the great influence of xenoestrogens. With too much estrogen relative to testosterone in their bodies, men lose body hair and develop problems with fat storage on their chests and hips. However, men sometimes walk around for years with unnoticed estrogen dominance; it doesn't result in the long string of painful discomfort and complaints that it does in women.

40+ WOMEN ARE EXTRA VULNERABLE

Women over 40 are especially vulnerable because from this age on, the hormone that strives to maintain a balance of estrogen—progesterone—declines. Normally estrogen also declines, so there's no problem. The decline of both estrogen and progesterone after the age of 40 is a normal process that shouldn't cause problems. But extra estrogen from external sources disrupts this balance. In addition, xenoestrogens have a powerful impact on your own estrogen, which is why they disrupt the balance even further. Also, being foreign substances, they are harder to break down and eliminate.

Estrogen Ensures Cell Division

Some of the issues that stem from estrogen dominance relate to cell division: fibroids, cysts, endometriosis, and tumors are tissues that do not belong in a woman's body.

Hundreds of studies have examined the relationship between the hormone-disrupting chemicals and cancer. These chemicals are viewed as one of two critical risk factors for breast cancer.[4] Diet and lifestyle are the second most important factor. This is logical because through your diet, you have a lot of influence on your estrogen levels.

And through your diet, you can ensure that the surplus of (xeno) estrogen is eliminated.

Xenoestrogens Are Hard to Excrete

Your body is typically well prepared to excrete a surplus of the body's estrogens as well as some of the external xenoestrogens. But your body is not built to handle an overdose of xenoestrogens, because it's difficult to get them back out. Breakdown and excretion can be arduous and require a lot of energy and nutrients. If your body has trouble excreting the xenoestrogens, it will store them in your fat cells to protect you.

AVOID XENOESTROGENS AND
INCREASE THEIR EXCRETION

On the one hand, it's important to avoid xenoestrogens as much as possible, and on the other hand, reliable excretion of them is equally important. That way your body will automatically decide to clear away your fat cells, which will no longer be required for safe xeno-estrogen storage. By means of your diet, you can help your body to break down and dispose of an overabundance of estrogen.

....

Xenoestrogens can be stored in your fat cells for decades, which is one of the reasons losing weight can be extremely difficult for women.

....

AROMATASE INHIBITORS: REDUCING THE CONVERSION OF TESTOSTERONE INTO EVEN MORE ESTROGEN

The downside of having too much estrogen in your body is that it's too much relative not only to progesterone but also to testosterone.

Female testosterone helps you build muscle and burn fat, gives you a healthy skin tone, and increases your sex drive. Strength training helps to build testosterone in your body, so that's definitely a good plan. Choosing food that inhibits the aromatase enzyme can also help. Aromatase can be found in your subcutaneous fat tissue and allows for conversion of testosterone to estrogen. And we certainly don't want that. The diet suggestions outlined in the Nutrition Compass include plenty of aromatase inhibitors.

TIPS FOR EXCESS ESTROGEN

EAT PLENTY OF FRESH GREEN VEGETABLES AND SPROUTS.

The chlorophyll in green vegetables helps your liver excrete and neutralize xenoestrogens. Strive for a pound of vegetables per day, half of them green and half raw. Cruciferous vegetables (all kinds of cabbage, broccoli, radish, arugula, cress, and brussels sprouts) in particular contain a chemical called DIM, diindolylmethane, which helps excrete a surplus of estrogen. Broccoli is excellent. DIM is also sold as a supplement.

EAT PLENTY OF FIBER.

Used estrogens should be excreted by your intestines. Fiber in your diet makes for good intestinal flora, which help your intestines with excretion. Healthy fibers are found, among other things, in vegetables, fruit, flaxseed, psyllium husks, coconut meal, oat bran, and legumes. Consider prunes too.

AVOID NONORGANIC MEAT, FISH, AND DAIRY PRODUCTS.

All factory-farmed meat, fish, and dairy is polluted with several chemicals. Avoid them as much as possible. More on this in Chapter 8.

CONSUME ALCOHOL WITH CAUTION.

Alcohol can increase your estrogen levels. In addition, alcohol means extra work for your liver, which you need for excreting surplus estrogens.

REDUCE YOUR DAILY EXPOSURE TO XENOESTROGENS.

Everything you breathe in or spray or spread on your skin is used by your body. Choose personal care products, perfume, cosmetics, and household products that are 100 percent natural or as natural as possible. Replace the pill with another form of birth control—the pill contains a large dose of synthetic hormones.

DRINK LEMON OR GRAPEFRUIT WATER.

Every morning, squeeze lemon or grapefruit into two large glasses of water; lemon and grapefruit are powerful aromatase inhibitors. (Read the information leaflets that come with any medications you take to find out if you can eat grapefruit.)

INSUFFICIENT PROGESTERONE

Progesterone is the second important female hormone that is mainly created by your ovaries, during the second half of your cycle. The production of this hormone declines after age 40. After menopause, the production of progesterone is taken over by your adrenal glands and your brain. Few women suffer from excess progesterone; progesterone deficiency is more common.

Progesterone Makes for Rest and Relaxation

Progesterone is, along with its importance in fertility and pregnancy, also the hormone that gives you a sense of peace. If your body creates the right amount of progesterone, you'll find it easier to relax and to feel cheerful. It has a positive impact on your sleep. In addition, progesterone helps your thyroid function, regulates your mucous membranes, lowers blood pressure, helps regulate body temperature, and promotes the burning of body fat. This is a hormone to stay friends with!

Unfortunately, your body often produces too little of it—too little relative to estrogen, that is, because they should be in balance.

Symptoms of Low Progesterone

Symptoms that may indicate a deficiency of progesterone are:
- all kinds of premenstrual complaints
- painful, swollen breasts
- irregular menstrual cycle
- heavy bleeding
- painful menstruation
- premenstrual fluid retention
- sleep problems
- anxiety attacks

Insufficient progesterone also automatically means excess estrogen, so the list of symptoms of estrogen dominance can also signal a progesterone shortage. It's always about the relative ratio between these two hormones. So what causes your body to create too little progesterone?

Cause #1: No Egg, No Follicle, No Progesterone

If you aren't yet in menopause, most of your progesterone is created by your ovaries. During ovulation, each mature egg sheds its follicle, now called the corpus luteum, and this corpus luteum is the main producer of progesterone. This is how estrogen and progesterone are kept in balance. In your 30s, progesterone production begins to drop, and as early as ten years before menopause, ovulation can also decline. If no egg matures one month, no progesterone is created that month either: no egg, no follicle, no progesterone! Since you have a period whether an egg has matured or not, you won't know this has happened. After months where no egg matures, a progesterone deficiency may develop. This isn't necessarily a problem unless you want to get pregnant. Lower levels of progesterone and estrogen in your 30s don't have to result in annoying symptoms if your body is otherwise in balance hormonally: it's working exactly as nature intended.

....

Progesterone is the basic building material of the stress hormone cortisol. With prolonged stress, cortisol consumes your progesterone, disrupting your hormone balance.

....

Cause #2: Cortisol Steals Your Progesterone

There's another reason progesterone can decline unnaturally and an imbalance can arise. Progesterone is the building material of the stress hormone cortisol, which your body creates automatically during stressful times. Your body is programmed to survive. As soon as it has to choose between the stress hormone cortisol and the soothing hormone progesterone, it will always opt for cortisol. That can save your life! But your body doesn't know you aren't really in mortal danger when you're watching a thriller, have an important exam coming up, are at the dentist, or are eating a fast-food meal full of additives. Your body just knows that it feels stressed, so it produces cortisol in case it's needed. The more soothing progesterone pulls the short straw, again and again.

STRESS AFTER 40 IS ASKING FOR TROUBLE

If you're a woman over 40, stress means an extra attack on your health. Your ovaries are naturally already producing less progesterone. Your adrenal glands must partly take over this task. During prolonged stress, however, your adrenal glands turn progesterone into cortisol, causing progesterone to drop even further. If you also have quantities of xenoestrogens wandering around in your body, then you'll expect the long string of health problems that I mentioned as connected to estrogen dominance and progesterone deficiency. These are two sides of the same coin. If you think too much stress could be causing your progesterone deficiency, read the tips about cortisol (pages 83 and 86).

Cause #3: Candida Infections Eat Progesterone

A candida infection—a proliferation of yeast in your gut, vagina, or both—can lower your progesterone level quite a lot. With a proper diet you can fight a candida infection. Take good care of your gut and your immune system, and candida will have little chance with you. See the tips for healthy intestines (page 113).

Your Thyroid Needs Progesterone

You also need enough progesterone for your thyroid to function properly. Now that you know this, you might not be surprised to learn that a quarter of women over 40 experience thyroid problems. Often prolonged periods of stress before 40 result in progesterone having drawn the short straw far too often.

TIPS FOR LOW PROGESTERONE

INCREASE YOUR VITAMIN C INTAKE.

Your adrenal glands need plenty of vitamin C to produce cortisol and progesterone, so eat plenty of fruits and vegetables. You could increase your intake of vitamin C–rich superfoods, such as acerola (Barbados cherry) and camu camu. These come in powder form and can be added to a smoothie. You can also take a vitamin C supplement.

REDUCE CAFFEINE AND ALCOHOL.

Caffeine and alcohol provide a direct serving of extra cortisol to your body, and therefore reduce progesterone. Try to avoid them as much as possible.

TRY VITEX (A.K.A. VITEX AGNUS-CASTUS, MONK'S PEPPER, CHASTEBERRY).

This herb can be found as a supplement. Vitex has been used for thousands of years for PMS and infertility complaints. Fifty years of scientific research show that vitex helps increase progesterone.[5] (Get advice from an expert—a lot of what's on the market is hardly effective or not at all.)

GET PLENTY OF RELAXATION AND REST.

It's hard to reduce stress in your life, but you can often provide an alternative: more rest. Nourish yourself with meditation, mindfulness, yoga, walking, soothing breathing exercises, a bath, or a hobby you enjoy. Anything that helps to reduce your stress is a bonus.

FOLLOW THE NUTRITION COMPASS.

The Nutrition Compass points you in the right direction to create a diet with the minimum of chemicals that add stress to your body.

REMEMBER THIS

- Your hormones work together: if one is out of balance, often others are too. It's smart to tackle them all at the same time.
- Disruption of the balance between estrogen and progesterone can result in many physical and mental issues and is common.
- Chemicals and stress can seriously disrupt this balance. Avoid both: prevention is better than treatment.
- Nutrition can have a positive impact on your estrogen level and thus on your estrogen–progesterone balance. It's important to keep your blood sugar (glucose) level as stable as possible.

MACA MAGIC

Maca is a superfood when it comes to balancing female hormones. It improves your body's balance by stimulating your hormone production. The drawback is that it doesn't really taste good. I often incorporate it into magical, tasty smoothies full of other goodies.

Almonds are an excellent source of easily absorbable calcium. Raw cacao is regarded as one of the most nutritious foods in the world, the richest source of magnesium, and a supplier of powerful antioxidants. Hempseed is an excellent source of vegetable protein, good for your arteries and memory. Add to that a date, which is a source of silicon (or silica)—important for your joints. Make your smoothie with Ceylon cinnamon and your blood sugar remains in balance. I often have this delicious drink as a substitute for a cup of coffee.

Here's What You Need
1 soft date
1 cup almond milk
1 teaspoon raw cacao
1 teaspoon maca
1 teaspoon shelled hemp seeds
6 pieces of frozen ripe banana
¼ teaspoon Ceylon cinnamon
a dash of Celtic Sea salt

Here's How You Make It
Remove the pit and cut the date in small pieces. If you use a dried date, soak it first in hot water for a few minutes. Put everything in your blender and mix well. Sip slowly and enjoy. This is power food!

2. INSULIN: WORKING OVERTIME

We ask insulin to do a huge job. Everyone, not only women, makes insulin. Its function is to make sure that energy is carried to your brain and muscles. Your body needs it all the time, even when you're sleeping.

Your body constantly uses energy. Fortunately, there are many ways you can give it an energy boost. Nutrition is a big one. Energy from what you consume arrives in your bloodstream via your intestines. Your blood glucose level, also called blood sugar level, rises.

At the words "blood sugar," you might tend to think only of sugar—white sugar, icing sugar... This is why I prefer the term *glucose*, to indicate that there are many more things than sugar that can increase blood glucose level.

....

Keeping your blood glucose level
stable is perhaps the most important strategy
for a healthy hormone balance.

....

WHAT IS INSULIN?

Insulin Carries Glucose to Your Cells

A high level of blood glucose is not healthy for your body because it disrupts all kinds of processes and can cause a lot of inflammation. Your body wants this level to get back to normal as soon as possible. In addition, that energy has to be carried to the cells of your muscles or brain, because these are the only places that benefit from it. As soon as your blood glucose level rises, your pancreas gets the signal to produce the hormone insulin. Insulin takes the glucose to your body cells. On arrival of the insulin, they open up and the glucose is absorbed into the cells. So insulin can be seen as the key to opening the doors of your cells.

Surplus Glucose Goes to Your Fat Cells

Excess glucose is stored in your muscle and liver cells, where it can quickly be made available. If after that you still have a surplus of glucose, it's stored in your fat cells as inventory for lean times—lean times that in our society don't often occur.

THE MANY ROADS TO HIGH BLOOD GLUCOSE

Your glucose levels don't rise only if you've eaten sweets. Refined carbohydrates such as white rice, white pasta, and white bread behave in your body in the exact same way as sugar. That's why they sometimes get called "fast" carbs: they cause a fast increase in your blood glucose because their grains have been stripped of their fiber. Also quickly increasing blood glucose are starches, including potatoes and other tubers and cereals, but also milk, all of which result in the production of insulin. And sugars are hidden in 80 percent of all supermarket products. You see in this table how often insulin is called to action?

Blood Glucose Levels Rise Quickly From:	Blood Glucose Levels Drop From:
All forms of sugar, including hidden	Insulin
Ingredients in "light" products	Insulin
Bad carbohydrates	Insulin
Milk sugars	Insulin
Starches	Insulin
Coffee	Insulin
Alcohol	Insulin
Cereals	Insulin

Blood Glucose Levels Rise Quickly From:	Blood Glucose Levels Drop From:
Chemicals in food	Insulin
Stress	Insulin
Eating too much	Insulin

It's important to remember that there are many ways to increase blood sugar but there is only one way it returns to normal levels: insulin. Insulin is a protective weapon that you have to use sparingly.

WITH INSULIN IN YOUR BLOODSTREAM, YOUR BODY CAN'T BURN FAT

At breakfast in a hotel I once heard a woman say to her friend that she had stopped eating sugar. Then she stuck a cheese croissant in her mouth. Next to her plate she had a glass of milk, a glass of juice, and a cup of black coffee. I thought, *Wow! Good thing you stopped with sugars, but insulin doesn't care whether you eat that breakfast or a large piece of cake. Your insulin is already working overtime.*

Most women stop eating sugar because they want to lose weight. That's a good idea, but unfortunately not enough. The annoying thing is that if insulin is circulating in your bloodstream, your body won't burn fat. Instead it will use the easily available form of glucose circulating in your blood.

IS IT ANY WONDER THAT LOSING WEIGHT IS HARD?

Have you noticed how many products in the left column of that table are addicting? We haven't made it easy for ourselves in our society. We humans are built for scarcity, but we live in paradise, with a large side of stress. No wonder obesity and diabetes have become severe problems. But if you know how your body works, you have the most important tools in hand to prevent both, and even to heal.

Too Many Highs, Too Many Lows

If your body produces too much insulin too often, then at some point your cells will become "deaf" to insulin and absorb less glucose. They get slowly worn out by all those times they open to absorb glucose. Because your body still wants to lower your dangerously high blood glucose levels, your pancreas produces extra insulin. This extra dose of insulin sends your blood sugar level suddenly into a valley, as your cells absorb the glucose. A dip in your blood glucose level doesn't feel good: you feel limp, maybe shivery or woozy; you can't think straight and you may develop a bad headache. You might have a panic attack or feel anxious or stressed. If your blood glucose peaks often, chances are you'll also often find yourself in a valley. These are times when your body sends you on the path to search for food because it wants to protect you by giving you energy.

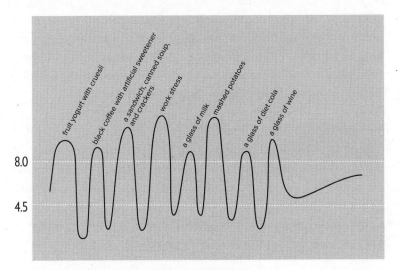

FLUCTUATING BLOOD SUGAR AND YOUR DIET

FLUCTUATING BLOOD SUGAR IS DEAD TIRING

In the Netherlands, we call it the "lunch dip": after a lunch that includes a few bread slices and a glass of milk, your blood sugar level spikes, then hits a valley. It seems as if the energy in your body disappears. A cup of coffee helps temporarily, but often the dip returns around four o'clock, when many women would lick the wallpaper if it were made of sugar. In short: fluctuating blood glucose is not only unhealthy but also dead tiring.

Cravings Aren't from Lack of Willpower

Are you personally acquainted with the phenomenon that if you start the day with something sweet, you continue to crave sweets all day? You're not the only one. Biologically speaking, there's no such thing as willpower; cravings have nothing to do with that. If your blood glucose level is too low, your body sends you looking for food. That's your survival mechanism doing its job.

Insulin Resistance Is a Forerunner of Diabetes

If the period of "cell deafness" lasts too long, the risk arises that you'll retain too much insulin in your blood even when your blood glucose is at a normal level. This is called *insulin resistance*, and if you do nothing about it, it's the precursor to diabetes. It then becomes almost impossible to lose weight, no matter what you do. This can be a very frustrating period, but fortunately it's reversible.

....

With insulin resistance, where too much
insulin continually circulates in your bloodstream,
it is next to impossible to lose weight.

....

CHRONIC MEANS "LONG-TERM," NOT "ETERNAL"

The word *chronic* means "long-term," not "eternal." Because we treat the symptoms but not the cause of many chronic diseases, including type 2 diabetes, we have slowly come to believe that a chronic disease is one you'll never get rid of. But this isn't always the case. Most chronic diseases can disappear if you get to the root of the problem. If your smoke alarm goes off, you don't take the batteries out to stop the noise—you search for the fire and put it out.

SYMPTOMS OF INSULIN RESISTANCE

Symptoms of (imminent) insulin resistance include:
- uncontrollable desire for sweets or fast carbs (such as bread)
- persistent obesity despite not overeating
- energy fluctuations
- food cravings throughout the day
- unwellness after not eating for a while (headaches, moodiness)
- tiredness after a meal
- a growing spare tire around the waist despite exercising
- irregular menstruation

TYPE 2 DIABETES: TOO MANY SWEETS?

Eventually, your pancreas becomes exhausted from producing all that insulin and throws in the towel. In the past this was the diabetes that only the elderly struggled with, but nowadays more and more young people, even children, have to deal with it. Having to produce too much insulin too often is the main cause of this, and you've already seen that it's not just the result of eating too many sweets.

Could Diabetes Be Tied to Chemicals?

More and more scientific evidence suggests that there's a connection between chemical exposure and the development of diabetes. A 2006 study examined the relationship between diabetes and the quantity of persistent organic pollutants (POPS) in the bodies of adult Americans. POPS are toxic substances that cannot be broken down; if the body can't properly dispose of them, they are stored in fat cells. The result was alarming: the higher the amount of these substances in the body, the greater the chance of diabetes.[6] Those most exposed to POPS were almost 40 times as likely to have diabetes. Since then many follow-up studies have unequivocally established the connection between certain POPS and diabetes.[7] If you are insulin resistant or have diabetes and want to get rid of it, examine the chemicals in your environment and strive to replace them with less harmful ones.

EXCESS INSULIN CAUSES HORMONAL CHAOS

Too much insulin in your blood results in hormonal chaos, as it means many other hormones cannot do their jobs properly. Everything in your body is disrupted by having too much insulin in your blood for too long. Have you ever noticed that if you eat candy or a plate of leftover spaghetti late at night you sleep badly? Insulin disrupts the production of the sleep hormone melatonin, which makes it hard to fall asleep. It also disrupts the production of the hormone DHEA, or dehydroepiandrosterone, and growth hormone, two that you need for vitality into old age. But the main problem is that it allows for chronic inflammation that may eventually lead to a range of chronic diseases.

Conclusion: Keep Your Blood Glucose Level as Stable as Possible

Keeping your blood glucose level stable is crucial for your vitality and health. By changing your diet, avoiding stress, and being more physically active, you can make sure your blood glucose levels are stable. That would look something like this:

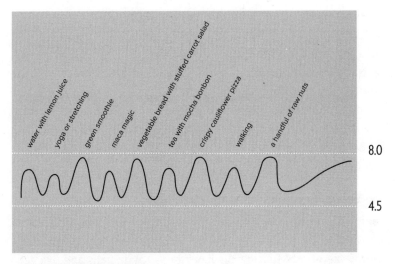

A STABLE BLOOD SUGAR LEVEL

MEASURING YOUR OWN GLUCOSE LEVELS

Are you wondering what *your* glucose levels look like during the day? You can measure this easily using a glucose meter, which you can order online or buy at a pharmacy. Test at different times throughout the day. Start early in the morning before eating, then before each meal and one to two hours after each meal. Understanding your blood sugar levels will give you important information about your health. If you're always between 4.5 and 8, congratulations! If you have bigger peaks and valleys, look at my tips about insulin (page 74).

HOW AND WHERE IN YOUR BODY IS ENERGY PRODUCED?

I imagine there are times you'd like some quick energy. When you have an important meeting or your grandchildren are visiting for the day, it's very tempting to grab an energy drink or some sweets. Still, raising your blood glucose isn't the right way to get that quick energy. This is because it's not just you that needs energy—your body also needs it, for all the work it does for you. Where does your body get that energy?

The Energy Factories in Your Cells

Energy is created in all your billions of cells, in energy factories called *mitochondria*. Each cell in your body contains many or a few of these energy factories. Muscle cells have a lot—brain cells and eye cells too—but abdominal fat cells have hardly any. In each muscle cell of an elite athlete, there can be up to 1,000! Remember this: the more energy factories you have, the more energy you will experience. No wonder top athletes with lots of muscles often have a lot of energy while overweight people often have considerably less—the latter have a lot of cells without energy factories.

DO YOU WANT MORE ENERGY? BUILD MORE MUSCLE!

Exercising and building more muscle mass is a really good way to get more energy. I speak from personal experience: three months after I started strength training, I could really feel that I had a lot more energy during the day. I can tell you, that absolutely stimulated my resolve to continue.

What your mitochondria need to continually give energy are the usable digested remnants of the food you eat. All the food you eat is broken down in your gut and split into usable and unusable particles. Your body excretes the unusable particles, while the usable particles are transported via your bloodstream to your liver and from there to all those trillions of energy factories.

The useful parts of your digested foods are your actual energy providers. They fuel your body to perform all its functions: old cell cleanup, healthy new cell creation, heartbeat, blood circulation, respiration, digestion, blood pressure regulation, hormone balance, and, on top of that, making sure that you can focus at that meeting and remain cheerful when your grandchildren trash the living room.

....

A healthy diet of vitamins, minerals, trace elements, and all those other invisible and unknown substances—these are your actual energy sources!

....

The energy boost you get from a piece of cake, a slice of pizza, a cup of strong coffee, or a bag of candy is only short-term. What your body really needs for ongoing high energy levels are the nutrients that you can find only in real food.

THE SMART SHORTCUT TO REMOVING GLUCOSE WITHOUT INSULIN

Have you eaten too many sweets or been too stressed? Get your body in motion! Walk up and down ten flights of stairs, go for a bike ride, wash a large window, or skip rope. Work your muscles! By using your muscles, you consume extra glucose and reduce the glucose peak. In addition, during physical activity your muscle cells directly absorb glucose without the intervention of insulin, and they continue to do so for up to two hours afterward. Physical activity is your main tool against developing insulin resistance.

The points of the Nutrition Compass will show you how to maintain a stable blood sugar level without having to eliminate all sweets or your daily cup of coffee from your diet.

TIPS TO AVOID EXCESS INSULIN AND INSULIN RESISTANCE

EAT A POUND OF VEGETABLES A DAY.

The best thing you can give your body as a counterpart to your sugar dips is anything that helps it produce real energy. Start by eating plenty of vegetables, in all the colors of the rainbow. Fermented vegetables are excellent because they also help build up your intestinal flora, which has suffered from too many sweets. Consider sauerkraut. Mixing vegetables with salt and storing them in a sealed jar creates a bacterial fermentation process that's very healthy for your intestines.

EAT HEMPSEED, QUINOA, AND ORGANIC EGGS.

Sugar addiction is best tackled with good vegetable proteins, which are the building blocks for dopamine and serotonin. Your body will use these neurotransmitters to create good feelings without sugar involved.

USE FISH OIL, KRILL OIL, OR ALGAL OIL.

These omega-3 fatty acids make your cells more sensitive to insulin.

REDUCE SWEETS AND BAD CARBS, AND ADD CINNAMON.

No matter how hard this is, try to get out from under the spell of sweets. Reduce it step by step. Add cinnamon wherever you can, because cinnamon helps keep your blood sugar levels more stable. Don't replace sugar with "light" products, which will lead you from the frying pan into the fire. Read more about this in Chapter 9.

DRINK AND EAT AS LITTLE AS POSSIBLE FROM TINS OR CARDBOARD PACKAGING.

There could be many pollutants in your food. Start by avoiding, as much as possible, canned food or cardboard with a plastic lining that contains the hormone disruptor BPA (bisphenol A). Glass is an excellent packaging material.

GET ACTIVE, PREFERABLY IN THE MORNING BEFORE BREAKFAST.

If there's one thing that will increase your metabolism and help to balance your blood sugar level, it's this: physical activity in the morning on an empty stomach, before breakfast. Your metabolism will remain high for several hours, so this is a very effective way to lose weight. Start by walking briskly enough to make you sweat for two minutes, alternating with three minutes of walking more slowly.

REMEMBER THIS

- There are many reasons why your blood sugar levels can rise. Insulin is the only hormone that can lower your blood sugar, and is therefore often deployed.
- Too frequent a need for insulin can lead to insulin resistance and type 2 diabetes.
- With insulin in your blood, your body cannot burn fat; insulin is sometimes called the "fat storage hormone."
- Keeping your blood glucose level stable is a key strategy for healthy hormone balance. You have a lot of influence on this through your diet.
- Being active is the most important tool in maintaining a balanced blood sugar level and preventing insulin resistance.

CRISPY SWEET POTATO AND PARSNIP FRIES

You don't have to avoid all sweet things once you become mindful of maintaining a stable blood sugar level. Sweet potato is definitely sweet, but it won't give your blood sugar an exaggerated peak and it provides for some healthy intestinal flora. Eat it together with a variety of vegetables.

You can use this simple recipe to roast many other kinds of vegetables. Consider pumpkin, celeriac, beetroot, cauliflower, onions, radishes, Jerusalem artichoke, and carrots. It's simple! Discover the convenience of roasting vegetables in your oven, and your life will never be the same. Oven roast a selection of vegetables, serve with a rich green salad including some legumes and a tasty dressing, and you have a complete meal. Vary the spices and herbs. For a crunchy effect, I sometimes sprinkle the vegetables with cornmeal (polenta or maize meal).

Here's What You Need

1 large sweet potato

1 large parsnip

1 tablespoon coconut oil

1 teaspoon cinnamon

2 teaspoons cumin seeds

1 teaspoon cumin powder

1 tablespoon cornmeal (optional)

a sprinkle of Celtic Sea salt

Here's How You Make It

Preheat the oven to 350°F. Line a baking sheet with ungreased parchment paper. Peel the sweet potato and parsnip, and julienne them (cut them into french fry–shaped strips). Put them in a large bowl and add the remaining ingredients. Toss together well. Spread them out on the baking sheet, slide that into the oven, and roast the vegetables for about 20 minutes.

3. CORTISOL: OUT OF CONTROL

Now we come to the wild alpha male of your hormones: the stress hormone cortisol. Cortisol is produced by your adrenal glands, mainly when your body has to spring into action. Your gut and brain can also create small amounts of cortisol. This is the hormone that makes you wake up in the morning and determines your circadian (night and day) rhythm; you need cortisol every day to function properly. If you're in danger, your body makes extra adrenaline and cortisol. These are great partners when you really need them. Cortisol also helps you if you need to write an exam or give a lecture to a large audience. A normal daily dose of cortisol is fine; an overdose of it over a long period of time destroys your body.

HEALTH AND STRESS NEVER GO TOGETHER

For you as a woman, stress is probably the biggest disruptor of your hormonal balance and hence of your health. Health and long-term stress never go together well for women. Cortisol can be a runaway train. Too much cortisol is the start of a whole avalanche to other problems. It is said that 95 percent of all health issues and diseases stem from or are aggravated by excessive stress. The list of symptoms associated with high cortisol seems endless. And as you have seen, stress is also a major disruptor of your blood glucose level.

> No healthy diet can
> beat prolonged stress.

There are stories about mothers who, in a dire emergency, were able to lift a car because their child was underneath it. That's the power of these stress hormones! But you pay a price for it, because if your body has to produce them for too long, your hormone balance will end up seriously disrupted.

Long-Term Stress and Your Thyroid

Cortisol is produced by your adrenal glands. If your adrenal glands have to continuously create a lot of it, they can suddenly become exhausted. To protect your adrenal glands, your thyroid may decide to slow your metabolism down to force you to take it easy. If you combat the symptoms of an underactive thyroid gland with medication, you don't address the root cause. Many women derive no benefit from these drugs. Giving your adrenal glands a rest is better advice.

Cortisol Robs You of Dopamine and Serotonin

After a long period of stress, there may come a time when you have both too much and too little cortisol. In the morning you might feel rushed (too much cortisol), in the afternoon exhausted (too little cortisol), or the other way around. A little stress is fine, but if your stress is not under control, that's not good. Stress also robs you of serotonin and dopamine, neurotransmitters that produce feelings of enjoyment, bliss, and motivation.

....

If you don't feel real joy or gladness
anymore and life is all a bit blah, beware: you
may have suffered from stress for too long.

....

STRESS HAS MANY HIDDEN FACES

You probably know if there's too much stress in your life, although many women discount the impact of stress too easily. I had a client who told me that she didn't really get stressed. It turned out that six months earlier she'd been thrown off a horse and spent two weeks in hospital. She was still in pain every day. Her daughter had anorexia and her husband's job was threatened. She worked more than 40 hours a week. But stress? No, she didn't really have any... Often women are so used to high levels of stress for years that they sincerely no longer know what it feels like to really relax.

Are you somewhere between 40 and 60? Then you belong to the first generation of women who worked full-time and also had full responsibility for running a household in a world that is increasingly stressful. The changes around us are happening fast. Nothing seems sure anymore, and many people experience the world as unsafe. And feeling like you aren't safe causes stress.

Stress Can Hide Anywhere

We can become so accustomed to high levels of stress that we no longer feel it. And that stress doesn't come only from an excessive workload or money problems. For your body, sources of stress can be anywhere: poor diet, upset circadian rhythms due to shift work, a visit to the dentist, chemicals, daily traffic jams, medication, too much exercise, too little exercise, fear, sadness, powerlessness in a relationship, and, yes, even falling in love can cause stress. With prolonged stress, eventually everything feels stressful, even small things.

Each person reacts to stress in their own way. Common symptoms of too much stress are:

· sleep problems
· irritability
· feeling harried
· trouble focusing
· trouble losing weight
· overeating
· skipping meals
· frequent cravings for sweets, coffee, alcohol, or energy drinks

STRESSED WOMEN OFTEN EAT TOO MUCH

Research shows that women more often than men eat too much in response to stress, and make less healthy food choices.[8] That makes sense, because you're desperate for something that will temporarily make you feel good and give you energy. Addictive foods such as sweets, junk food, and coffee do this. Unfortunately, these foods will *not* make your body happy.

STRESS MAKES YOU FAT: HOW IT WORKS

Cortisol and sugar give you quick energy. As with sugar, cortisol ensures that glucose is made available quickly, in this case from your adrenal glands. Under acute stress, glucose will also be taken from the reserves in your muscles and liver. This increases your blood glucose level. The glucose is carried to your cells by insulin. Cortisol gives you energy to quickly take action. But if you don't run away fast or fight for your life, this boost of glucose won't be used and will instead be stored in your fat cells. Thus, excessive stress can make you fat.

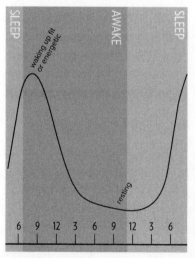

HEALTHY

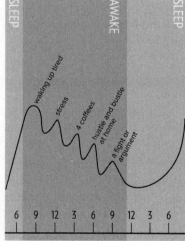

UNHEALTHY

Just like your blood sugar level, your cortisol level should remain relatively stable, not fluctuate too much. Cortisol raises not only your blood sugar level, but also your blood pressure. Like sugar, it can lead to chronic inflammation in your body.

Normally, cortisol peaks an hour after waking up and declines over the course of the day. Research shows that many women show a cortisol peak around five o'clock. That is the moment when they come home from work exhausted, their children or partner (or both!) wants their attention, and they have to get to work in the kitchen to cook supper. It would be worth building in a half hour of relaxation at this time.

HOW DOES YOUR WAIST BECOME A FAT MAGNET?

In women 40 and over, this is the ultimate recipe to increase your spare tire: eat and drink lots of processed foods, sweets, coffee, and/or alcohol and have a lot of stress. Your waist then becomes a magnet for fat! Make sure insulin and cortisol don't need to work overtime. That said, some women *lose* weight from excessive stress. Each body has its own survival strategy.

THE STRESS-REDUCTION HORMONE: OXYTOCIN

Stress reduction is crucial for your health and vitality over the long term, but reducing stress is more easily said than done because your common sense can't just make you not worry about that next exam or a son or daughter in trouble. It's not that simple. Cortisol is controlled by your so-called reptilian brain, over which you have very little say. It's your survival mechanism, the part of your brain that goes into action in the event of danger. In an acute emergency, your non-reptilian brain—your human brain—responds way too slowly.

Fortunately, there is a hormone that can reduce your stress and that you yourself can stimulate: oxytocin. Oxytocin is the hormone your body makes when you're breastfeeding, but also when you have sex and cuddle. If you're under a lot of stress, make sure you have something or someone to cuddle with or care about.

Lower Your Stress Level with a Chat

There is another way, and that's through conversation. As a woman, you can significantly decrease your stress level by chatting it away. Research shows that in women, but not in men, this leads to the production of significantly higher levels of oxytocin.[9] No wonder, then, that women are more in need of conversation than men! Work with your hormones and make sure you have a group of girlfriends around you who help you reduce your stress just by listening to you. I didn't know this fact, but for decades it had been my strategy to destress by talking—calling a friend and having a good venting session. I always feel more relaxed and relieved afterward. Now I understand why: oxytocin!

What Helps You to Relax?

Everything you find fun and relaxing can help reduce your stress level: meditating, walking in nature, yoga, swimming, gardening, sculpting, massage, coloring for adults... it doesn't matter what it is. Make sure you have something in your life that provides relaxation and fun, and enjoy it with gusto! You don't drive your car around on an empty tank: you refuel while you can still drive to the gas station. Refuel yourself in time too. If you can't do this on your own, find help in the form of a stress coach. Too much stress can be produced just in your thoughts. If you learn to see them only as thoughts and worry about them less, you're already winning.

PLAN 15 MINUTES A WEEK TO WORRY

I received a golden tip from a stress coach, a tip I use regularly. At the time, I was worried about my financial situation, because I was considering quitting my job and starting my own business. But in my head I was always hearing that little voice saying, "Yes, but…" My coach advised me to set aside 15 minutes a week for this voice and to ignore it the rest of the week. On Friday, between a quarter to five and five o'clock, I gave this little voice all the space it needed and listened obediently to all its objections to me quitting my job. If the voice piped up during the rest of the week, I said, "No, you can only talk on Friday, at a quarter to five," then ignored it. It took practice, but because of this I've learned not to let myself be carried away by fearful thoughts that keep me small.

Stress and sugar look very much alike in your body.

TIPS FOR A FLUCTUATING CORTISOL LEVEL

STRIVE, AS MUCH AS POSSIBLE, FOR A STABLE BLOOD SUGAR LEVEL.

Cortisol raises your blood sugar levels. Sometimes you can (temporarily) do nothing about that, but use nutrition to keep it as stable as possible.

INCREASE YOUR VITAMIN C INTAKE.

Support your adrenal glands with vitamin C. Eat plenty of fresh fruit and vegetables. You can increase your vitamin C intake with superfoods such as camu camu and acerola berry. These come in powder form and can be added to a smoothie.

INCREASE YOUR INTAKE OF OMEGA-3 FATTY ACIDS.

Research shows that omega-3 fatty acids help to reduce cortisol. Sources include flaxseed and walnuts. You also get a hefty boost from fish oil, krill oil, or algal oil. Read Chapter 7 for more information.

GO EASY ON COFFEE, CHOCOLATE, ENERGY DRINKS, AND ALCOHOL.

These raise your cortisol level even more. Replace them, as much as possible, with green, white, or herbal tea, nondairy milk, or hot water with ginger.

SOME HERBS CAN HELP YOU TO REDUCE YOUR CORTISOL.

Try rhodiola to lower cortisol, and valerian or sage (*Salvia officinalis*) to help you relax.

GET PLENTY OF OXYTOCIN.

Give yourself an overdose of cuddling, sex, and conversation.

BREATHE.

Your breathing is a wonderful way to influence stress. By inhaling in shorter breaths than you exhale, you can relax your nervous system. Breathe quietly into your belly for two beats in, two beats out, then take a two-count rest. Do this for a few minutes. Put your hands on your stomach so that you can feel it rise and fall. You can even do this at work, or in the bathroom!

TAKE AN EVENING BATH WITH MAGNESIUM SALTS.

Stress consumes a lot magnesium. Use a supplement or take frequent warm baths with magnesium flakes (Epsom salts). Add a soothing scent such as lavender. Magnesium helps you relax. Dive right into your bed afterward, and you'll sleep like a baby.

ADRENAL FATIGUE: WHEN THE TRAIN COMES TO A STOP

If you have a lot of long-term stress, you can end up exhausted. Your adrenal glands can simply quit sooner or later due to years of working overtime. If your adrenal glands are depleted, they produce very little cortisol. This is called burnout, and you can then literally feel physically, mentally, and emotionally burned out. I speak from experience. It's as if your exhausted body has given up control of the steering wheel of your life and put the car in park. Willpower has no effect and your brain has completely lost its way.

Could Exhausted Adrenal Glands Cause Menopause Symptoms?

Many women arrive at menopause with adrenal fatigue. This could explain why so many nowadays experience severe menopause symptoms. Unfortunately, few doctors can recognize adrenal fatigue, so keep good track of the amount of stress in your own life. Your adrenal glands not only are an important key for your hormone balance, but also control the amount of joy and pleasure you feel in your life. Would you like to measure your cortisol level? Many natural health practitioners and doctors can administer a cortisol saliva test.

Adrenal fatigue is usually the result of years of doing too much for others but not enough for yourself. Recovery requires a multi-faceted approach: physical and mental and emotional.

When it comes to your diet, the Nutrition Compass is, in my personal experience, the fastest direction-setter to recovery. With the Nutrition Compass you will, on the one hand, give your body the nutrients it needs and, on the other, eliminate stress and hormone disruptors from your diet as much as possible. This is an excellent beginning. Seek out professional help in the form of a coach, stress counselor, or orthomolecular therapist if you think you need it. You don't have to do it all alone. You really don't!

TIPS FOR LOW CORTISOL

INCREASE YOUR VITAMIN C INTAKE.

As for a fluctuating cortisol level, support your adrenal glands with vitamin C. Eat plenty of fresh fruit and vegetables. You can also add superfoods such as camu camu and acerola berry, which come in powder form and can be added to a smoothie. Choose red and purple fruit above all.

DRINK LICORICE TEA AND EAT GRAPEFRUIT.

Research shows that both can help increase your cortisol level.[10] Keep an eye on your blood pressure; licorice can increase it. Read the information leaflets that come with your medications to determine if you can eat grapefruit.

TRY ASHWAGANDHA AND MACA.

Ashwagandha is the most commonly used herb in Ayurvedic medicine; it can support your adrenal glands. Maca can help get your hormones back in balance.

EAT SIX TIMES A DAY.

Too little cortisol can lead to binge eating. It's better to eat a little bit six times a day at fixed times than to eat a lot three times a day. Focus especially on healthy fats, sprouts, vegetable protein, and fiber; eat more of these than you're used to. Be careful with sweets and fast carbs—they worsen adrenal problems.

TAKE A GOOD MULTIVITAMIN AND MINERAL SUPPLEMENT.

Stress has depleted your body, creating a shortage of all kinds of vitamins and minerals. Fill it with a good orthomolecular multivitamin that includes the important B vitamins.

WANT LESS FOR A WHILE.

Give in to your need for peace and relaxation and take good care of yourself. Your body needs it.

REMEMBER THIS

- Next to fluctuating blood glucose levels, stress is the largest disruptor of your female hormonal balance and hence your health.
- Stress has many faces; your body can be stressed without you noticing it or feeling stressed out.
- Oxytocin may help you to reduce stress; sex, cuddling, and conversation help to reduce cortisol.
- Get plenty of rest and relaxation to counterbalance stress. Seek professional help if you find this hard. No matter how healthy your diet is, the effect of too much stress is hard to counteract.

CHILLED FRUIT SOUP WITH EXTRA VITAMIN C

Red and purple fruits such as blueberries, raspberries, strawberries, blackberries, and pomegranate seeds are full of antioxidants and other cancer-preventing substances. They are also powerful aromatase inhibitors that help keep your testosterone–estrogen balance in equilibrium. To give your adrenal glands extra support, try this soup, with its boost of camu camu and acerola or acai powder—superfoods that provide high doses of vitamin C. During my burnout, I ate this soup a lot.

An easy way to make a smoothie with vegetable protein is to add a spoonful of nut or seed butter. My favorites are almond butter, cashew butter, and tahini, a sesame paste. They give your smoothie a full, creamy taste. Don't leave them out: you need the fats to slow down your digestive system, to absorb the vitamins and minerals more readily, and to help you feel full longer.

Here's What You Need

1 cup mixed red and/or purple frozen summer fruit
½ cup coconut water
1 cup spinach or other green leafy vegetables
1 rounded teaspoon of almond paste
¼ teaspoon Ceylon cinnamon
1 rounded teaspoon of acai powder, acerola powder, or camu camu (optional)

Here's How You Make It

Let the fruit thaw for about 10 minutes. Put everything in your blender and blend until thick and creamy. Pour into a wide mug. Sprinkle with Energetic Woman's Granola (page 45). Eat the soup slowly with a spoon.

4. THYROID HORMONES:
TESTING ISN'T KNOWING

Every second, your hormones are adapting to your environment to keep you alive. Your thyroid gland is particularly sensitive to what's happening inside and outside your body. Women have larger thyroid glands than men, with the result that we're more sensitive to our environment. In our society, this does not seem to be in our favor. Some women suffer from an overactive thyroid gland, but an underactive thyroid is more common. Thyroid hormone stimulates the metabolism by setting the mitochondria, the trillions of energy factories in all your cells, to work. It is therefore very important to look after your thyroid in order to protect your health and energy levels.

SYMPTOMS OF AN UNDERACTIVE THYROID

The symptoms you may experience when there's something wrong with your thyroid hormones are diverse because the thyroid has such a big influence on your body. They range from extreme fatigue to dry skin, hair loss (also your eyebrows), weak nails, constipation, and water retention; from persistent inflammation, muscle spasms, joint problems, and cold hands and feet to heart rhythm disorders, weight gain without obvious cause, persistent obesity, poor concentration, reduced memory, fibromyalgia, depression, and sleep problems… and that's not even all of them. These symptoms may also occur even when nothing is wrong with your thyroid, because something is out of balance elsewhere.

If your thyroid hormones work well, you have energy, you can think clearly, and you're cheerful. Your thyroid hormones are your physical, mental, and emotional battery charger.

MENOPAUSE OR THYROID PROBLEMS?

In the United States, 24 percent of women over the age of 42 are on thyroid medication and 11 percent on antidepressants. Mary Shomon, who has studied thyroid problems like no other, has called menopause the "thyropause." It's the period in which your energy levels, moods, and weight can change dramatically because your body produces less estrogen and progesterone in combination with excess cortisol, all of which have their effect on the functioning of thyroid hormones.

WHEN IT COMES TO YOUR THYROID, TESTING ISN'T KNOWING

The functions of thyroid hormones are complex and often not well understood. Problems may arise in different parts of your body. From one tiny part of your brain, your pituitary gland, your thyroid receives the command to produce thyroid hormones. This signal is TSH (thyroid-stimulating hormone). Your thyroid then creates the hormone thyroxine (also called thyronine, or T4). However, it's not T4 that's active in your body but another hormone, T3 (triiodothyronine). T3 is created when T4 is converted using substances that include progesterone from your liver and from other cells in your body. For proper thyroid function, you need, among other things, sufficient progesterone, because T3 is the only active thyroid hormone controlling your entire metabolism—the processing of your nutrients, cell renewal, and waste removal. There are a lot of steps to all this, and a lot can go wrong along the way.

Diagnosing Women's Thyroid Problems

A quarter of all women over 40 deal with the symptoms of an underactive thyroid. This is 20 times higher than in men. Many women live with thyroid problems without knowing it, or are told that nothing is wrong when in fact there is. A doctor often just checks to see if the thyroid gland itself is working properly, and a problem in the conversion to active, free T3 is overlooked. Therefore, it's important to look not only at the amount of TSH and T4, but also at the amount of free T3 that your body creates.

A thyroid can also slow down as a result of an autoimmune disorder, such as Hashimoto's disease. It is therefore important to check if your body is producing thyroid peroxidase (TPO) antibodies, which may indicate an autoimmune disease. Insist on your doctor referring you for this test; many doctors are ill informed about the latest findings concerning thyroid problems. Without testing for TSH, T4, free T3 levels, *and* the production of antibodies, you and your doctor won't know exactly what is going on. Always look for the cause—don't just fight the symptoms. Also be aware that an underactive thyroid is not always indicated in a blood test.

STRESS AND THE UNDERACTIVE THYROID

Stress has a significant influence on your thyroid. When you're under a lot of stress, the stress hormone cortisol consumes a lot of your progesterone. Because of this, there's less progesterone available to ensure the conversion of T4 to T3. Your thyroid gland itself works fine—you don't have an underactive thyroid—but you have *symptoms* of an underactive thyroid because the T4 to T3 conversion isn't going well.

Your Thyroid Can Slow Down to Protect You

Your thyroid can slow down as a result of the depletion of your adrenal hormones. The slowing of your thyroid gland also slows your metabolism, thereby protecting your body against further overload. In effect, your thyroid throws the brake on your overloaded body. An underactive thyroid may be your body's clever protective mechanism!

In 50 percent of cases of thyroid dysfunction, there are also over-burdened adrenal glands. Instead of listening to our bodies and slowing down for a while, we take drugs to keep our thyroid gland going (even though our thyroid is often not the root of the problem!) and keep chugging along. Chances are that sooner or later we will pay the price in the form of other, serious health problems.

You often see that the thyroid gland slows down in cases of chronic inflammation, and there's a link to insulin resistance and estrogen dominance as well. Then the question is which is the result and which the cause.

....

You can have the symptoms of an underactive thyroid even when there is nothing wrong with your thyroid.

....

THE PILL AND YOUR THYROID

Unfortunately, the contraceptive pill can also have a negative impact on the function of your thyroid. Use of the pill can result in a shortage of important nutrients that your thyroid needs, such as magnesium, selenium, zinc, and the critical B vitamins. The pill also takes its toll on your liver, which is where its synthetic hormones are broken down. If you have thyroid problems, you should ideally use a form of birth control other than the pill.

HORMONE DISRUPTORS AND YOUR THYROID

Hormone disruptors don't just hamper the proper function of your estrogens: they can also disrupt thyroid hormone function. The

150 chemicals known to disrupt your thyroid include PCBs (polychlorinated biphenyls), dioxin, and BPA (bisphenol A).[11] They can have an effect on both the thyroid gland itself and on levels of free T3. One substance we frequently ingest is BPA, found in the soft plastic layer on the inside of the cans and cardboard of our packaged food. Given the increase in thyroid problems in women, it seems advisable to avoid these substances as much as possible. Also avoid heavy metals such as mercury (oily fish can be contaminated), fluoride in toothpaste, chlorine, and bromine, all of which can cause thyroid problems.

TIPS FOR SYMPTOMS OF AN UNDERACTIVE THYROID

ADD IODINE.

A healthy thyroid needs iodine among other nutrients. Iodine is found in organic eggs, white fish, samphire (glasswort or sea asparagus), seaweed, algae, and iodized salt. (Note: This advice does not apply to all autoimmune disorders of the thyroid gland—too much iodine can sometimes work against you.)

EAT A FEW RAW BRAZIL NUTS EVERY DAY.

Brazil nuts contain selenium, and your body needs selenium for the conversion of T4 to T3. Buy them as fresh as possible and keep them in the refrigerator.

AVOID GLUTEN AS MUCH AS POSSIBLE.

Celiac disease, an intolerance of gluten, triples the incidence of the symptoms of an underactive thyroid. Gluten can damage your intestinal wall, impeding your body's absorption of the nutrients it needs for a healthily functioning thyroid. There is Italian research that shows that gluten-free food can counteract the symptoms of an underactive thyroid.[12] (You can get gluten-free pasta even in Italy these days!)

SKIP THE CARB-FREE DIET.

To lose weight, many women avoid all carbohydrates. However, your body needs carbohydrates to ensure the smooth conversion of T4 to T3, so don't avoid them all.

CHOOSE A TOOTHPASTE WITHOUT FLUORIDE.

Hundreds of studies show a relationship between the use of fluoride and thyroid problems.[13]

BE CAREFUL WITH UNFERMENTED SOY PRODUCTS.

Soy contains goitrogens, substances that disrupt the production of thyroid hormones by interfering with the thyroid gland's iodine uptake.

REDUCE STRESS.

Make sure cortisol is not robbing you of progesterone, and fit plenty of relaxation into your schedule.

REMEMBER THIS

- One quarter of women over 40 experience the symptoms of an underactive thyroid.
- We usually talk about an underactive thyroid, but there's often actually something going on not with the thyroid itself but with the function of various thyroid hormones.
- Proper testing for thyroid hormone levels is critical to understand what exactly is going on.
- Hormone disruptors can negatively impact your thyroid and your thyroid hormones. As much as possible, avoid food that comes in plastic, cans, and cardboard packaging lined with a thin layer of plastic.

CHICKPEA AND GREENS SALAD
WITH TAMARI BRAZIL NUTS

I like taking this salad to a barbecue. Don't wait too long to serve yourself because the bowl empties quickly!

I add Brazil nuts especially for the thyroid. Hempseed is a complete protein. That's good for everyone at the barbecue who prefers (like me) to eat fruits and vegetables instead of a lot of meat or fish. Tamari is salty soy sauce that does not contain wheat.

Here's What You Need

½ cup Brazil nuts

a splash of tamari

½ cup pumpkin seeds

about 8 cups of a mix of torn soft green leafy vegetables, such as
 lamb's lettuce, watercress, or spinach

1 cup cooked chickpeas (if using canned chickpeas for convenience,
 choose a brand packaged in a glass jar)

1 cup pineapple pieces

½ cup shelled hemp seeds

a dash of Celtic Sea salt

For the dressing

3 tablespoons plus 1 teaspoon olive oil

1 teaspoon curry powder

1 teaspoon turmeric powder

juice of ½ lemon

1 teaspoon fresh ginger, grated

1 teaspoon raw honey

Here's How You Make It

Chop each Brazil nut into three or four pieces. Roast the pieces briefly in an ungreased frying pan on high stovetop heat until they are light brown. Remove the pan from the heat and pour the tamari over it. Stir until the nuts are evenly coated in tamari. Pour them into a large bowl and let cool. Roast the pumpkin seeds in a clean, dry frying pan until they pop and are light brown. Add them to the Brazil nuts and also cool. Then add the remaining salad ingredients and toss everything together. Put all dressing ingredients in an empty glass jar, tighten lid and shake well. Taste to make sure you have the right balance of acid and sweet. Finally, toss the dressing with the salad and serve.

5. LEPTIN AND GHRELIN: FEEL FULL WHEN YOU SHOULD

Leptin and ghrelin are like estrogen and progesterone: hormones that belong together. They too must be in balance with each other. In a healthy woman's body, they both get to work when needed. Ghrelin is the hormone that sends you signals about hunger; it arouses your appetite. This hormone is primarily created in your stomach. Its counterpart, leptin, is also called the "satiation" hormone: it gives you a timely warning that you've eaten enough.

DO YOU HAVE ENOUGH LEPTIN?

When you're eating, leptin is the hormone that gives you the message, on time, "Thank you so much—I've had enough." This hormone is primarily produced by your fat cells. If you rarely get this signal (except if you've eaten so much that you're *really* full), chances are you have a deficit in leptin.

You could draw the conclusion from this that overweight people should automatically feel satiated faster, since they have more fat cells—more fat cells, more leptin production. This might seem logical, because why would you need so much food if your body has enough fat storage? This is exactly as nature intended, but the normal, healthy function of leptin and ghrelin has been disrupted in our society. There's also a link between the disruption of these two hormones and an underactive thyroid, so it's particularly important for women to factor these two hormones into their overall hormonal balance.

LEPTIN RESISTANCE: WHEN YOUR CELLS ARE DEAF TO "I'VE HAD ENOUGH"

It must be obvious that most women wrestle with a lack of leptin, or, rather, with leptin resistance. If your body has produced an abundance of leptin for any of a host of reasons—for example, if you're overweight—your cells will end up deaf to its signals. This works the same as insulin resistance. If you're overweight, with a body mass index of 25 or more, you will no longer receive the signal that you've eaten enough. Because of this, you're in an unhealthy vicious circle: you don't get the signal that you've eaten too much, so chances are you eat more than you need to; as a result, you gain more weight, resulting in even fewer signals that you've eaten enough. Almost all women who are overweight are leptin resistant but tormenting themselves with the idea that they have no willpower to stop eating. It's never a matter of willpower. I'll say it again: it's your hormones! Leptin resistance can cause persistent obesity.

Women Are More Leptin Resistant Than Men

As women, we are unfortunately more leptin resistant than men because we have more fat cells than men. Even a slim woman can be leptin resistant. In slim women, the fat cells are not so much on the outside as on the inside—in particular, between the organs in the abdomen. This means that you have too many fat cells compared to your muscle mass. Indeed, working out to increase muscle mass is an excellent idea.

Insufficient leptin not only is an important cause of overeating, but also plays a major role in (auto)immune diseases and all sorts of hidden inflammation underlying a wide range of chronic diseases.

So what's the main cause of all this leptin misery?

FRUCTOSE, OR FRUIT SUGAR: SOUNDS INNOCENT BUT IT ISN'T

For leptin to function well in your body, a low triglyceride level is needed. Triglycerides are small particles of fat in your bloodstream. You need some, but not too much. Junk food, processed foods, bad carbs, and all sugars, particularly fructose, will increase the level of triglycerides in your bloodstream. If you have too many triglycerides in your blood, leptin's signal to your brain that you've eaten enough will be blocked. The only way to safely reboot your body's awareness of satiation is to reduce the number of triglycerides in your blood. This can be done by avoiding all sweets, fast carbs, and processed foods—but mainly fructose—as much as possible.

Fruit Keeps Getting Sweeter

Fructose is a sweetener found naturally in fresh and dried fruit and in other natural products such as honey and agave. This natural form of fructose is usually not the main problem, but it's still wise to be cautious. Many women who want to eat healthier replace unhealthy processed sweets with a lot of sweet fruit or dried fruit. This is a step in the right direction, but please be aware that our fruit gets sweeter every year. Did you know that kiwis were originally sour fruits? And apples and oranges were not nearly as sweet as they are now. The crossbreeding and modification of fruit is making it sweeter. In addition, compared with 50 years ago, we consume more fructose-laden food and drinks. Eating two pieces of fruit per day with all their fibers is healthy, but juicing and drinking five oranges is asking for a fructose/glucose boost.

....

Around 1900 we ate 15 grams of
fructose per day. Now we eat around 65 grams.

....

If you have excess weight, problems with your blood sugar, or diabetes, please be careful with sweet fruit until your body is back in balance. It's preferable to choose more sour fruits such as berries, sour apples, pomegranates, grapefruit, and lemons.

HOW MUCH FRUCTOSE IS IN THAT SUGAR-FREE BOX?

Ironically, most foods for diabetics are sweetened with fructose, because fructose causes blood sugar levels to increase more slowly than glucose. But that does not make these products healthy. Avoid sugar-free products at the grocery store, whether you're diabetic or not.

Fructose Attacks Healthy Livers

The biggest problem, however, is not the fruit in your fruit bowl. The biggest problem with fructose is that it, in combination with glucose, is found in virtually all (approximately 80 percent of) processed food products, including savory products like tomato ketchup and peanut butter. There's no fruit involved: this fructose is made from corn. It's cheap, very sweet, and easy to add to all kinds of products. Unlike glucose, fructose cannot, however, be regulated by insulin and stored as reserve inventory in your muscles and fat cells. Fructose goes directly to your liver, where it is converted to fatty acids, including the triglycerides that are found in your blood. Excess fructose is converted into fat in your liver. This can result in fatty liver disease, even at a young age. You may not notice any issues right away, but a fatty liver has difficulty carrying out all its functions. In time, this can cause liver inflammation and other liver diseases.

Fructose: The Fastest Route to Aging

Fatty liver is just one of the consequences of fructose: fructose is also referred to as the fastest route to aging.
- An excess of fructose disrupts your sense of satiation, leading to overeating and all the frustrations of extra pounds.
- Are you addicted to sweets? Chances are it's a fructose addiction.

- If you have problems with your blood glucose level, this is likely a fructose problem.
- If you have problems with your cholesterol, this is probably also a fructose problem.
- Fructose is, to a large extent, the underlying cause of excess belly fat, obesity, and diabetes.
- Fructose increases uric acid, which leads to problems such as gout, kidney stones, and arthritis.
- More and more people are experiencing abdominal pain as the result of excessive fructose intake. Unexplained abdominal pain can be the result of a fructose intolerance. This is similar to a lactose intolerance: the enzyme that helps absorb fructose in the small intestine no longer functions normally. Because of this, a (large) portion of the fructose you consume ends up in the colon, where the intestinal bacteria quickly ferment it, causing abdominal pain, bloating, and flatulence.

HFCS: A WOLF IN SHEEP'S CLOTHING

HFCS, or high-fructose corn syrup, is a powerful synthetic sweetener composed mainly of fructose. It is made from corn and is therefore cheap. HFCS is used in many of the processed food industry's products instead of regular sugars. You'll see HFCS listed as corn syrup, fructose syrup, glucose-fructose, fruit sugar, or natural sugar.

Fructose Intolerance Can Cause Depression

In her book Gut: *The Inside Story of Our Body's Most Underrated Organ,* Giulia Enders writes that the medical world has recently acknowledged that unnoticed fructose intolerance can cause depression. In our digestive system, the amino acid tryptophan likes to attach itself to fructose. If we can't absorb most of the fructose, we defecate the tryptophan and fructose together, unused. But tryptophan is the raw material of serotonin, the feel-good hormone.

Leptin Resistance and Your Thyroid

If you ingest too much processed food (full of sugars, fast carbs, and fructose), the hormone leptin will increase in your body. A high leptin level sends a signal to your brain to slow your metabolism down by impeding your thyroid function. If you are leptin resistant this happens constantly, as there is always too much leptin in your body. Leptin resistance can therefore affect the healthy functioning of your thyroid. Do you need more reasons to pay attention to how much fructose you consume?

SLEEP CAN HELP LEPTIN BALANCE

For every hour you don't sleep, you produce 5 percent more ghrelin and 5 percent less leptin. Insufficient sleep makes you hungry. An important tool to get your leptin levels back into balance is to ensure a stable day-and-night rhythm and get plenty of sleep. By that I mean seven to nine (!) hours of healthy, deep sleep. Women need more sleep than men. Go to bed and get up at fixed times, and don't adjust your times too much on weekends. Avoid the artificial light of your computer, television, LED lamps, and smartphone during the last hour of the day. Create a cool, dark bedroom. Don't eat sweets, carbohydrates, or junk food in the few hours before you go to bed. This disturbs the production of the sleep hormone melatonin.

TIPS FOR LEPTIN DEFICIENCY AND RESISTANCE

DON'T EAT TOO MUCH.

There's nothing as delicious as the satisfied feeling after a healthy meal when you know you didn't eat too much. There's a relationship between leptin resistance and insulin resistance, so check the tips for too much insulin (page 74) too.

EAT PROTEIN AND HEALTHY FATS FOR BREAKFAST.

Avoid any form of sweet foods (including fruit) as much as possible in the morning, and eat proteins in the form of eggs, savory pancakes, or green smoothies. Avocados are an excellent choice!

ADD ENOUGH OMEGA-3 FATS.

Omega-3 is your best friend when it comes to counteracting leptin resistance. Eat fatty fish, walnuts, and flaxseed. Use supplements as such as krill oil or algal oil.

EAT ENOUGH AT EACH MEAL, AND AVOID SNACKS.

Leptin resistance often results in between-meal cravings. Try to break this habit. Eat a little more at each meal (especially healthy fats and proteins), and avoid snacks. If your leptin is restored, you'll no longer have cravings between meals.

AVOID SWEET DRINKS.

Avoid, as much as possible, sweet beverages, especially sodas, fruit juices, energy drinks, and alcohol. Many drinks are sweetened with high-fructose corn syrup, under many different names. Avoid them. Alcohol also contains sugar and means an extra tax on your liver.

GET ACTIVE.

Intense exercise isn't urgently needed, but physical activity is. Research shows that overweight women have more cravings if they exercise intensely than men do. If you're overweight, focus first on sitting less and getting more general physical activity. Take a walk, for example, or go cycling. Make sure you sit for no longer than 60 minutes at a time, then stand up and move around for a few minutes.

GET ENOUGH GOOD-QUALITY SLEEP.

Turn off your television or computer in good time. Take a long, hot bath with magnesium flakes (Epsom salts) and soothing oil (lavender). Read a nice book and get to bed on time.

REMEMBER THIS

- Leptin is the hormone that gives you a sense of feeling full.
- Leptin works well when there are few triglycerides in your body. Processed foods, fast carbs, and all sugars, especially fructose, cause an increase in triglyceride levels.
- Fructose is found in 80 percent of all processed foods. It is hidden behind innocent-sounding names like "fruit sugars" and "natural sugars."
- Too much fructose leads to fatty liver and a host of other health problems, including weight gain and obesity.

GREEN VEGETABLE MINI-OMELETS

These vegetable mini-omelets are ideal for breakfast if you want to control your blood sugar and don't want sweets for breakfast. They're also delicious for lunch.

An egg contains vitamins A, E, D, K, and B12. If you eat little meat, fish, and dairy, eggs are an important source of B12, which is found only in animal products. Eggs also contain iron, zinc, selenium, and folic acid, four important minerals for women's health. Always buy organic eggs: the nutritional value is much lower in nonorganic ones.

You can make these mini-omelets with different vegetables, so adapt this recipe creatively. Be sure to choose vegetables that cook fast, such as finely chopped leek, peas, and small tomatoes. This is my favorite version. You can omit the feta, but it makes the omelets extra delicious!

Here's What You Need (for 6 servings)

1 cup grated zucchini
1 cup spinach, finely chopped
15 fresh basil leaves, cut
   into strips
2½ ounces of feta, in
   small pieces

1 tablespoon mixed herbs
freshly ground pepper and
   Celtic Sea salt
3 eggs

Here's How You Make It

Put all the vegetables, the feta, and the spices in a large bowl. In another bowl, beat the eggs well. Add to the vegetables and stir together. Heat a large frying pan and pour a generous splash of olive oil in it. Scoop three piles of the vegetable mixture into the pan and press them flat with a spatula. Cook a few minutes on each side. Make sure the egg is cooked through. Keep warm in the oven if you are not serving immediately.

6. YOUR GUT: THE HEART
OF YOUR HEALTH

A healthy hormone balance for you as a woman is not possible without two important organs: your gut and your liver.

Health begins in your gut, because if your gut doesn't function properly, your whole body is affected, including your endocrine system. Your intestinal flora consists of trillions of good and bad bacteria, which together weigh only about four and a half pounds, or two kilos. You need both the good and the bad, but it's important to keep the good bacteria in the majority. This reduces your risk of being overweight and of getting all sorts of nasty diseases. You do this by feeding your healthy intestinal bacteria—literally. Through good nutrition, of course.

At least 20 different hormones are created in healthy intestines. These hormones affect not only your physical health but also your mental and emotional health. How you feel and behave is to a large extent determined by the bacteria in your gut.

EXPENSIVE POO: MALNOURISHMENT ON A HEALTHY DIET

Your guts are where the nutrients from your food are absorbed into your body. All the food you eat is broken down into small packets of useful vitamins, minerals, and thousands of other substances in your gut. These packets pass via your blood through your liver, where they are checked for toxic substances, and then these thousands of nutrients feed all the cells in your body.

If your gut doesn't function properly, these packets of nutrients may not be well absorbed. And no matter how healthy your diet is, a large part of the valuable nutrients may remain unused. I call this expensive poo. Meanwhile, your cells don't get the nutrition they need and slowly your body becomes malnourished. This affects all your hormones and your overall health and can cause all sorts of often misunderstood symptoms.

LEAKY GUT: SMALL HOLES BETWEEN
YOUR OUTER AND INNER WORLDS

Your intestinal wall makes the important distinction between what can be absorbed by your body and what is unceremoniously sent, unused, to the exit. Your small intestine is permeable, but only for very small packets of nutrients. Its wall is lined with the intestinal mucosa: the gatekeeper to your blood. This contains all kinds of enzymes that make sure the food particles are small enough to pass through. Keep in mind that food is always foreign matter to your body, whether you accidentally swallow a rubber cap or consciously eat a strawberry. Your gut determines what your body will absorb and what it won't.

Serious problems arise if your intestinal mucosa becomes inflamed or damaged. Your intestinal wall can develop holes, similar to what can happen to a bicycle tire; there are then leaks from your intestine to your blood. These holes can admit all kinds of bacteria, toxins, parasites, and food molecules into your bloodstream, none of which belong there. Then your immune system works overtime to throw these intruders out, and it becomes overloaded. In addition, your hormonal balance can be disrupted.

We call this phenomenon a "permeable" or "leaky" gut, and it's usually the beginning of a lot of misery. One problem is that you don't feel like you have a leaky gut because it doesn't hurt. As a result, it's often overlooked. It doesn't help that many mainstream doctors don't know about this phenomenon.

When Foreign Substances Get in Your Blood

Because these foreign substances in your blood can come from anywhere in your body, the symptoms that may arise from a leaky gut are very diverse.

Think, among other things, of:
· all kinds of skin problems—eczema, hives, psoriasis
· irritable bowel syndrome (IBS)

- long-term fatigue
- heartburn
- allergic reactions
- joint problems
- fibromyalgia
- concentration problems and bad memory
- all kinds of autoimmune diseases, including thyroid problems
- depression and mood swings

....

Over a third of all people with
depression also have a leaky gut.

....

Skin problems such as eczema and psoriasis are often a result of
a leaky gut, because your body is still trying to get rid of the dirty
substances through your skin: your skin is a detox organ. Applying
something to heal damaged skin is pointless—you aren't getting rid
of the cause.

The Immune System in Your Gut

Eighty percent of your immune system is in your colon. A leaky gut
can affect your immune system, causing autoimmune diseases. Autoimmune diseases are much more common in women than in men,
so taking good care of your gut is especially essential for women.

WOMEN ARE PARTICULARLY AFFECTED BY AUTOIMMUNE DISORDERS

Autoimmune disorders are in the top 10 causes of death of women
up to age 65 and, in the United States, are the second most important cause of chronic diseases—multiple sclerosis, type 1 diabetes,
rheumatoid arthritis, Crohn's disease, Graves' disease, Addison's

disease, systemic lupus, and many more. The epidemic of auto-immune disorders is growing but it is not known why. A link to intestinal health has apparently not yet been made.

The Main Causes of a Leaky Gut

This damage or inflammation of your intestinal mucosa comes from somewhere; something like that doesn't just happen. Common causes—we call these *allergens*—are:

· gluten
· added fructose
· sugars
· dairy products (especially from cow's milk)
· chemical additives in food, such as flavor enhancers (monosodium glutamate, or MSG, is one) and artificial colors, flavors, and fragrance
· chemicals that leak into food from packaging materials such as tin and plastic
· antibiotics in your diet (found in nonorganic meat, fish, or dairy)
· pesticides (found in nonorganic fruits and vegetables)
· alcohol
· stress
· medications such as antibiotics and anti-inflammatory drugs

Furthermore, a yeast infection or parasite in your intestine can also be the cause of a leaky gut. The yeast *Candida albicans* is one source that can proliferate in your system.

As you read the list above, you will realize that your normal daily diet includes many irritants. Your intestine can process small amounts of just about anything, but dealing with aggressive attacks every day is too much for even the strongest intestine. Realize too that with age, your resistance to these allergens diminishes. It may be that for years you had no problems with dairy, fructose, or gluten, so you're probably not inclined to link your skin problems, under-active thyroid, arthritis, Crohn's disease, or chronic fatigue to a gut that is finding it increasingly difficult to cope.

How to Fix a Leaky Gut

Happily, you can do a lot yourself to give a leaky gut the chance to recover. To start with, avoid all the aforementioned irritants as much as possible. If you have a strong suspicion that you have a leaky gut, avoid them for two weeks and watch how you feel. The cells of your intestinal lining can regenerate in seven days, but if you've had a leaky gut for years, this process will take longer. The degree to which your gut is permeable can vary, depending on how irritated your intestinal mucosa is and how long it's been irritated. Taking a good probiotic supplement can help: it will provide your gut with healthy intestinal bacteria. A wide variety of bacteria from natural, partly fermented foods, however, is better and cheaper.

HEALING YOURSELF

Because we all have different intestinal bacteria, one person can handle a certain food while another cannot. You might be able to eat strawberries without problems but your girlfriend gets an itchy rash from them. If you change your intestinal flora through your diet, you may also rid yourself of years of food allergies and even from an autoimmune disease. More and more women are not accepting the prognosis that they will never be free of their autoimmune disease. They largely heal themselves with their diet, or at least get their symptoms under control. Several women have written books about this. Search for Dr. Terry Wahls (multiple sclerosis), Meghan Telpner (Crohn's disease), Molly Vazquez (alopecia totalis), or Izabella Wentz (Hashimoto's disease).

YOUR GUT IS YOUR SECOND BRAIN

Did you know that 95 percent of the neurotransmitter serotonin, which gives you such good feelings, is created in your gut? The neurotransmitter dopamine and the important sleep hormone melatonin are also largely produced in your intestines. Your intestines' nervous system is just as rich and complex as your brain's, and your intestines, through your main nerve—the vagus nerve—are connected to your brain. Your brain and your intestinal flora constantly communicate with each other.

DEPRESSIVE BRAIN OR DEPRESSIVE INTESTINES?

Antidepressants are sometimes tested on mice left swimming in a bowl of water where they have nowhere to land—a hopeless situation. At some point, they give up and let themselves drift. If they're willing to continue to swim following the administration of antidepressants, scientists see this as a positive signal that the mice have "hope" longer, hope that they'll be okay. Depressed mice give up easily.

In 2011 neuroscientist John F. Cryan examined if he could influence the behavior of the mice with a dose of beneficial intestinal bacteria. He found that the mice with the revamped intestines swam longer and had lower stress hormone levels than the control group. The bacteria in their intestines worked very much like an antidepressant. According to Cryan, the mice behaved as if they had received antianxiety medication.[14]

Your Gut Determines Much of How You Feel

There's a reason why your intestines are called your second brain: they have great impact on your mood and emotions. You know that happy feeling when you've completely emptied your bowels? A cleared head certainly has a relationship with tidy intestines! We have always assumed that our emotions and our moods are all in our head and that they have no connection to the rest of our body. But more and more research indicates that our emotions and moods do in fact originate in our gut, not our head! Research shows that people with bowel problems such as irritable bowel syndrome and ulcerative colitis are more likely than average to suffer from depression and anxiety attacks, even if there is no apparent outside cause for either. It also works the other way around: the intestinal flora of people with Parkinson's disease has proved to be very different from that of healthy people.

....

Your intestinal health has a lot of influence on
both your physical and your mental health.

....

Your gut also plays an important role in your body's elimination of toxic substances, which in our society is becoming increasingly important. Avoiding toxic substances is not always possible, but increasing your resistance to them is!

In short, taking good care of your intestinal flora means taking care of your health and vitality. With your dietary choices, you have great influence on your intestinal flora. Just remember that your intestinal flora lives almost exclusively in your colon—the trick is to eat food that travels from your small intestine to arrive in your colon undigested. Otherwise, the bacteria will get nothing from it.

A diet that follows the points of the Nutrition Compass makes for good nutrition for you and all your gut flora friends.

ANTIBIOTICS CAUSE CHAOS IN YOUR GUT

Antibiotics are substances that fight bacterial infections caused by bacteria that have invaded your body and done damage. We call this *inflammation*. If your immune system is compromised, it's difficult for your body to fight infection by itself. Antibiotics can be found in nature—think of ginger, cinnamon, garlic, turmeric, and coconut oil—but sometimes natural sources are not enough. In some cases, such as with a serious pneumonia, powerful medications are required. The problem with antibiotics is that they don't distinguish between good and bad bacteria. This means that in your intestinal flora, both the good and the bad bacteria are killed. As a result, the bad bacteria can easily get the upper hand. This weakens your immune system, which in turn can cause all sorts of nasty new problems, including candida infection, which is common in women. If it really is necessary to follow a course of antibiotics, make sure you offset any damage with a course of strong probiotics.

TIPS FOR HEALTHY INTESTINES

EAT PLENTY OF VEGETABLES, SPROUTS, HERBS, AND LEGUMES.

These contain soluble fiber, which you need for good intestinal bacteria. Cereals can provide a helping of nonsoluble fiber.

EAT HEALTHY FATS.

In addition to plenty of fiber, your intestinal bacteria also need healthy fats. You can read more about healthy fats in Chapter 7.

DRINK PLENTY OF WATER, PREFERABLY FILTERED.

If you're going to eat more fiber, it's important to also drink more water; otherwise, you just end up with bowel problems. If possible, drink filtered water.

DRINK KEFIR OR EAT OTHER FERMENTED FOODS.

This will feed your intestines an extra helping of healthy bacteria. Ideally, make it yourself; factory-made food contains barely any probiotic bacteria.

AVOID SUGARS AND STRESS.

Bad gut bacteria feed on sugars. The more sugars you eat, the better the bacteria have it and the more trouble they cause. Eliminate sweets as much as possible. Under acute stress, your gut bacteria can become completely disrupted within 24 hours. Be aware of the relationship between stress and your gut.

AVOID TOO MUCH ANIMAL PROTEIN AND FATS.

In particular, avoid the products of nonorganically raised animals. Nonorganic animal protein and fats may contain antibiotics that you ingest indirectly.

GET ACTIVE.

Healthy bowels love physical activity. A largely sedentary lifestyle has a negative influence on your intestinal flora. Walking 10,000 steps a day is much better than going for a two-hour run only on the weekend.

REMEMBER THIS

- Your health begins in your intestines. If your microbiome isn't healthy, all sorts of health problems arise, both physical and mental.

- Certain substances can irritate your intestinal mucosa and result in a leaky gut, even though you may not feel it directly. Try to avoid these substances as much as possible.
- Ninety-five percent of the happiness hormone serotonin is created in your gut. There is, therefore, a relationship between your gut health and your mood.

SPICY SOUP FOR UNEXPECTED GUESTS

Lentils, like all legumes, contain plenty of fiber and are therefore very good for your intestines. The advantage of red lentils is that you don't need to soak them in advance. They also contain a lot of iron, which is always good for women.

This spicy soup, which you can have on the table in half an hour, is one of my favorites. I almost always have these ingredients in the house, so it's an ideal soup for unexpected guests. Nutrition from a can is not my preference. Fresh tomatoes are better, of course, but sometimes I opt for convenience and speed. Don't make it too hard on yourself in the kitchen.

Here's What You Need (for 4 servings)

1 tablespoon coconut oil

2 leeks, finely chopped (if you don't have leeks on hand, use onions instead)

4 cloves garlic, finely chopped

1 tablespoon finely chopped fresh ginger

1 tablespoon cumin powder

1 pinch cayenne pepper

1 cup red lentils

½ cup passata (sieved tomatoes) from a glass container

1 large can diced tomatoes (14 ounces)

3 slices of lemon

4½ cups vegetarian broth

fresh coriander

Here's How You Make It

Heat the coconut oil in a stockpot and add the finely chopped leeks. Sauté till soft. Add the garlic and ginger to the leeks together with the cumin powder and cayenne pepper. Rinse the red lentils well and add to the pot. Now add the passata, the can of diced tomatoes, the lemon slices, and the broth. Bring gently to a boil and let simmer for 20 minutes. Once the lentils are cooked, you can serve the soup. Finely chop a generous amount of coriander leaves and use to garnish each serving.

7. YOUR LIVER: THE INDISPENSABLE CLEANUP CREW

Your liver is very happy with healthy intestines, because if your intestines do not function properly, this means extra work for your liver. Your liver has 400 different functions, of which directly or indirectly maintaining your hormonal balance is a critical one. The list of complaints you can experience if your liver does not function properly is endless.

MEET YOUR HARD-WORKING LIVER

Job #1: Disposal of Used Hormones and Waste

You probably know that your liver is involved in all kinds of detoxification processes in your body. One important task for the liver is to convert waste, unusable substances, and toxic substances into harmless substances, after which they can be safely drained and excreted through your intestines and kidneys. Detoxification in the liver involves three steps: making the substances water soluble, rendering the toxins harmless, and disposing of them.

Not all waste and toxic substances can be avoided; some waste products result from normal processes in your body. Removing those won't normally be a problem for a healthy body. The body's own waste molecules are familiar to the body and can be broken down more easily than foreign molecules.

Toxic Substances Are Trickier to Remove

As your body is increasingly exposed to toxins from your environment, work for your liver becomes heavier. The antioxidants normally created by your liver to protect your cells against free radicals are also used to remove toxic substances. If your body can't fully detoxify them or if there are too many toxic substances, then this will eventually lead to all kinds of chronic diseases and premature aging.

A large portion of these toxic substances are the chemical hormone disruptors discussed earlier in this book. These substances have been developed to have long-lasting effects and are difficult for your body to break down. The more time and energy your liver must spend on neutralizing and disposing of these hormone disruptors, the less attention it can pay to all its other important functions.

HOW DO YOU MAKE LIFE EASIER FOR YOUR LIVER?

How do you make doing everything it needs to do as easy as possible for your liver? It takes two steps: prevention and plenty of nutrition.

Prevention Is Better Than Cleanup

The less clutter in your home, the less you have to clean up. This also applies to your body. Don't make this more difficult than necessary: try, as much as possible, to keep chemical hormone disruptors out of your life. I understand that you can't instantly stop taking medications you may need or quit a job that exposes you to a lot of chemicals, but starting today you can change your diet, personal care products, cosmetics, and household products and choose ones that are more liver friendly. From now on, whenever you can, choose products free of harmful chemicals, preferably 100 percent natural.

Nutrition, Nutrition, Nutrition

I'm going to explain something complicated but very important: the detoxification process. This is so important because it shows just how essential the right nutrition is for a woman's body if she's to remain healthy or get better. Will you try to stay with me?

The detoxification process follows three steps: first, take the toxic substances and make them water soluble; next, make the toxins harmless; and finally, dispose of them. This process must run through all three steps smoothly. Unfortunately, along the road there can be quite a few pitfalls because as the substances are made water soluble, they can be reabsorbed into your body or converted into other substances that are even more damaging. The detoxification process is a painstaking task for your liver.

In order for the detoxification process to run properly, your liver needs a wide range of nutrients—vitamins, minerals, amino acids, antioxidants, trace elements, salvestrols, and thousands more. These help your body produce enzymes needed for the entire detoxification process. The challenge is that to neutralize and break down each toxin, a separate combination of enzymes is needed. A shortage of any particular nutrient, such as iodine, zinc, or sulfur, could result in certain toxic substance not being disposed of by your body. Scientists don't yet know exactly which nutrients are needed to remove which toxic substances. Luckily, your body *does* know how to manage this challenge, and that is why it is so important to provide it the best possible support by eating the largest possible combination of different nutrients in as varied a diet as possible.

Detoxification happens in your body every second of the day and night. It's worth considering detoxing as a daily activity.

HOW XENOESTROGEN DISPOSAL WORKS

I'd like to expand on the elimination of xenoestrogens, which can so seriously disrupt a woman's body. Xenoestrogens cause persistent obesity and chronic diseases, and may eventually even lead to various forms of cancer, which illustrates the crucial importance of eating a wide variety of unprocessed, especially plant-based, foods.

Chlorophyll

To neutralize and dispose of xenoestrogens, first and foremost you need green vegetables. The chlorophyll from these green vegetables helps to make xenoestrogens water soluble, the first phase of detoxification. Algae, such as chlorella, spirulina, and marine phytoplankton, are another good source of chlorophyll. Chlorella also helps to remove heavy metals from your body. After being made water soluble, xenoestrogens are converted into three forms of estrogens. Two of these can still do damage, so it's important to neutralize and dispose of them. For this your liver needs various other substances.

DIM

DIM (diindolylmethane) is a phytochemical that helps convert the harmful chemicals into a harmless form. You can find DIM in the cruciferous family: broccoli, brussels sprouts, cauliflower, kale, cabbage, Chinese cabbage, arugula, radish, kohlrabi, and garden cress. These vegetables should be briefly heated for the DIM to be released. Stir-frying and steaming are better than boiling so you won't throw the DIM out with the water. Broccoli sprouts are excellent sources of DIM.

Calcium D-glucarate

Calcium D-glucarate is another substance that your liver needs to neutralize and excrete xenoestrogens. You'll find it in the cruciferous family and in legumes, pumpkin, melon, asparagus, avocado, oat flakes, apples, and apricots. Alfalfa sprouts are abundant in calcium D-glucarate.

Glutathione

Glutathione is the most important antioxidant in your body because it is involved in many processes. Lack of sufficient glutathione could be the basis of all kinds of hormonal issues. It is also the most important substance for the detoxification and removal of xenoestrogens and heavy metals. The forerunner of this substance is the amino acid cysteine. Both substances can be found in sulfur-rich foods such as soft-boiled eggs, avocado, cooked spinach, cooked brussels sprouts, walnuts, hazelnuts, almonds, figs, cooked chicken, and sunflower seeds. Lentil sprouts are one of the best sources. To produce enough glutathione, your body also needs plenty of vitamins B3, B6, B9, and B12, plus some selenium and magnesium.

You'll find B3 in nutritional yeast flakes, coriander, maca powder, and unprocessed rice bran. B6 you'll find in soft egg yolks, unprocessed rice bran, and all kinds of dried green herbs, such as chives, chervil, coriander, oregano, thyme, rosemary, and parsley. It's also present in spices like cayenne pepper, turmeric, curry, and paprika. B9 is also called *folic acid* or *folate*. You'll find it in a wide variety of raw, leafy green vegetables and herbs, and also in agar, nutritional yeast flakes, red beets, sesame seeds, and sun-dried tomatoes.

You can find plenty of B12 in meat, fish, and (organic) dairy, but it's not advisable to eat much of these if you want to keep your hormones in balance—more on this in Chapters 8 and 10. My favorite source of B12 is organic eggs, and I also take a sublingual tablet daily as a supplement. Selenium is especially important to help your liver reuse glutathione so that you don't have to continually produce it. Raw Brazil nuts are a good source of selenium. Eat them as fresh as possible. Magnesium is also needed but many women have a shortage of it because stress depletes magnesium stores. An excellent source of magnesium is seaweed. It can also be found in raw cacao, buckwheat, coriander leaves, poppy seeds, dried pumpkin seeds, and unprocessed rice bran.

YOUR BODY NEEDS A HUGE VARIETY OF NUTRIENTS

Do you get a picture of how important all these (mainly plant-based) foods are for your health, but also how much variety is needed? The same breakfast every day, such as a bowl of yogurt with granola, or the same lunch of four slices of bread with cheese, is a missed opportunity! Your body needs so many different nutrients, and you can't be endlessly eating. Therefore, as much as possible, vary everything you eat and regularly try new recipes with new ingredients.

....

Eating a wide variety of vegetables,
herbs, fruit, seeds, and nuts will almost automatically
provide you with over 10,000 different
nutrients. Many of these nutrients scientists don't
yet understand, but your body does!

....

Be aware that stress uses up many of these nutrients and that as a result your liver may not have enough of them left. If you're under a lot of stress, it can become very difficult for your liver to detoxify. And if your liver fails to eliminate toxic substances, your body will decide to store them in your fat cells. Avoid toxic substances in your environment as much as possible, especially if you're dealing with persistent obesity.

The good news is that your liver has huge self-healing abilities. This organ is so important! If you take care of your liver, it will recover and all its functions will work well again.

TIPS FOR A HEALTHY LIVER

CHOOSE CHEMICAL-FREE UNPROCESSED FOODS.

Eat "real" food as much as possible, preferably organic. All chemicals that enter your body must be disposed of by your liver.

EAT A WIDE VARIETY OF GREEN VEGETABLES.

Eat half your green veggies raw and the other half lightly cooked, ideally steamed. This will help your liver with the first step of the detoxification process. Learn to make green smoothies.

USE GREEN SUPPLEMENTS.

Try chlorella, spirulina, phytoplankton, and wheatgrass. These are good sources of chlorophyll.

EAT A WIDE VARIETY OF PLANT-BASED PRODUCTS.

The emphasis in your diet should be on variety—your liver needs many different phytochemicals. Grapefruit has a powerful effect on the detoxification properties of your liver. (Ask your pharmacist if your medications allow you to eat grapefruit; your liver's detoxification process is so powerful that it could also eliminate the medication.)

LIMIT COFFEE AND ALCOHOL.

Both coffee and alcohol create an extra burden on your liver.

FIND AN ALTERNATIVE TO THE PILL.

The pill contains a large dose of synthetic hormones, which your liver must neutralize and eliminate. Try a nonhormonal birth-control method.

REMEMBER THIS

- Your liver plays an essential role in the elimination of all kinds of used substances and toxins from your body.
- The first thing you can do for your liver is to avoid ingesting or coming in contact with toxic substances as much as possible.
- The second thing is to eat a wide variety of mainly plant-based foods, so that your body ingests as many different nutrients as possible to help the liver neutralize and eliminate toxic substances.

TURMERIC MILK

Turmeric is a spice that has been used in Chinese medicine for centuries. Turmeric contains curcumin, a chemical that is an anti-inflammatory, a strong antioxidant, and antibacterial, and that also seems to be toxic to tumor cells. Turmeric supports not only your gut but also your liver. "Let nutrition be your medicine" is certainly true for turmeric. Adding pepper increases the efficacy and stimulates your body to burn fat. Turmeric is a basic ingredient in curry. I often add extra turmeric to a curry dish. If I'm not feeling well or have an infection, I make a mug of turmeric milk.

Here's What You Need
1 teaspoon turmeric (preferably organic)
1 teaspoon maple syrup
a sprinkle of fresh pepper
1 cup nondairy milk (cashew nut milk is very tasty)

Here's How You Make It
Add the turmeric, maple syrup, and pepper to a mug. Preheat the nondairy milk gently in a pan, but do not boil. Put a small amount of the milk in your mug and stir until you have a smooth paste. Then add the rest of the milk and stir again. Sip slowly. It feels very nourishing—give it a try.

3

ARE YOU MALNOURISHED?

E VERYTHING IN YOUR body is interconnected. You can't consider an organ in isolation from the rest of your body. If your intestines aren't working properly, you're going to end up noticing this in your skin, and if your immune system isn't working properly, your brain will falter. That is why it is important to provide your entire body, including all its organs, with nutritious food, so that you can ensure optimal hormonal balance.

MALNOURISHED IN THE WESTERN WORLD

Malnourished in Terms of Nutrients

In my opinion, many women in Western society are malnourished. So are men and children. They're malnourished not in calories but in nutrients. I'm not the only one who thinks this; the Dutch Nutrition Center agrees with me. If you as a woman eat according to their guidelines, the food pyramid, then according to their 2011 report you'll still be deficient in six important nutrients: vitamin A, vitamin D, iron, selenium, folic acid, and zinc. Without these essential nutrients, it is impossible to get your hormones in balance and, over the longer term, to stay healthy and vital. Vitamin A, vitamin D, selenium, and zinc are essential nutrients to keep your thyroid healthy.

Interestingly, the Dutch Nutrition Center also indicates that 95 percent of Dutch people aren't following its guidelines and so probably have even more deficits in addition to the list of six that it suggests. It turns out that of adult women up to age 69, only 10 percent eat two pieces of fruit a day and only 5 percent eat the recommended 250 grams (just under 2 cups) of vegetables. So there is a good chance that your body, just like mine a few years ago, has become deficient in nutrients.

> You can't fix hormonal problems on your own. You can only feed your body so well that it starts fixing itself.

Our Hectic World Needs Powerful Nutrition

The Dutch Nutrition Center's advice has, in my opinion, been overtaken by the times. I am convinced that a 40+ woman would be short of nutrients even if she did eat according to their guidelines. The advice to women aged 40 to include 4 to 5 slices of bread, 4 to 5 servings of grains or potatoes and 2 to 3 servings of dairy food daily is, in my opinion, asking for health problems. In our hectic society with all its stress, our body requires a better and more varied diet!

Malnourished in One of the Richest Countries in the World

The Netherlands is one of the richest countries in the world, where all kinds of foods are readily available. However, in the Netherlands we are heading for 6 million chronically ill people, and the situation in other Western countries is not much better. A lot of the people in our Western world are too heavy and, at the same time, are malnourished, because often these go together.

MALNUTRITION HAS LED TO DISEASE FOR CENTURIES

That malnutrition leads to disease we know—we just have to look to our history. We can learn important lessons from the past.

Scurvy at Sea—A Lack of Exercise?

Scurvy was once the leading cause of death of the crews on sailing ships. In the medical world, it had long been believed that scurvy was a problem of blood circulation, caused by a lack of movement. But in 1747, British naval doctor James Lind discovered that sick men healed within six days if they ate two oranges and one lemon. Nobody knew exactly why.

It was not until 1865, after hundreds of deaths, that the British Board of Trade made it mandatory that lemon juice be a daily part of the menu on merchant ships. The nutrient that we now call vitamin C was discovered only in 1933.

Beriberi in the Rice Fields—An Infection?

At the end of the 19th century in the Dutch East Indies, thousands of people died suddenly due to a previously unknown illness called beriberi. Doctors thought it an infectious disease. Then Dutch physician Christiaan Eijkman discovered that chickens that ate mechanically husked white rice became ill but chickens that got brown rice did not. He drew the conclusion that white rice contained a toxic substance and the husk contained the antidote. It did not occur to him that people became ill as a result of a shortage of a nutrient. Later his assistant Gerrit Grijns did come to this conclusion, although he had no idea what nutrient it was.

This nutrient was isolated only in 1926 and was named vitamin B1, or thiamine. By the end of the 19th century rice-husking machines regularly stripped rice of this essential nutrient, with the result that a lot of poor people across Asia became ill and eventually died, as rice was their main food.

....

Filling your belly does not mean nourishment.

....

Why Couldn't Food Be a Cure?

Doctors and researchers have always overlooked that large groups of people became ill due to a lack of certain nutrients. To this day there are doctors and scientists who say that diet cannot cure because it is not scientifically proven.

....

Has the earth always been
round, or did it only become round
after scientists proved this?

....

If you can get sick due to a lack of nutrients, then can you be cured by adding these nutrients back to your menu? What do you think? Nutrients are important for all our cells and can make us sick or better.

NUTRITION IS INFORMATION FOR YOUR CELLS

A veterinarian can read the health of an animal from its coat. The fur reflects whether the animal is healthy or not. The same applies to us. If things haven't been going well for you for a long time, you'll see it in your skin, hair, and nails. If your body lacks certain nutrients, it will first supply what there is to your vital organs, such as your heart, lungs, and liver. If there are still some nutrients left, these will go to your skin, hair, and nails. "I'll survive without beautiful skin and hair," your survival mechanism thinks, "but not without a functioning heart and liver." Unfortunately, from the outside we can't see if your heart, liver, and lungs are getting the proper nutrition. I like to say, *Nutrition is information for all the cells in your body.* Everything you eat is continuously sending your cells all kinds of messages: produce this hormone, dispose of these old cells, convert this to protein, trigger these immune cells, switch on this gene, and so on. Food is so much more than just fuel!

What Information Does Your Body Need?

People are mammals. In my opinion, this should rob us of the arrogance of thinking we are superior and should put us back in our place of nature. The genetic difference between humans and chimpanzees is smaller than that between chimpanzees and gorillas, and a simple aphid seems to have the same number of genes as humans. In other words, we are not so very different.

We Ate What Nature Gave Us

For centuries, our ancestors reproduced themselves by eating what nature gave them. All over the world, nature determined what we ate. Usually this was a combination of plants, tubers, seeds, nuts, fruits, insects, eggs, fish and shellfish, seaweed, and meat. People are omnivores, which means that we can eat pretty much anything that nature gives us... fortunately.

Eighty percent of the Inuit diet consists of fish and meat due to lack of vegetation in their Arctic environment. The Maasai, a nomadic people from Africa, on the other hand, let their cows live. The traditional diet of the Maasai (along with plants, fruits, tubers, insects, and honey) consists largely of cow's milk and the blood of cows that is obtained from bloodletting.

Women Knew What to Do Naturally

Women worldwide determined what was put "on the table," and as a result we now have more than 7 billion people on our planet. Women have always known how to feed their families. They have never needed a scientist, nutritionist, dietitian, or food pyramid to do so. We humans are mammals from the wild. Everything provided by nature is recognized by the cells in our body. The cells of this food and our own cells speak the same language: our bodies can work with this.

A Warm Reception

Imagine the arrival hall of a big airport. As soon as people recognize their loved ones after a long separation, there are cheers, or at least a big smile and a hug. Something like this happens in your body when natural nutrients come in contact with your cells: a warm reception. It's what went wrong when we started to interfere with the products nature made for us. When an apple became an apple pie manufactured to stay fresh for three weeks.

A MALNOURISHED BODY BEGS FOR NUTRIENTS

A body that is malnourished will continue to whine for real, nutritious food. This is partly the cause of the many "unexplained" cravings for women, who say they have no emotional reason to lapse into binges yet their body forcefully sends them to the fridge. It's your body in survival mode that sends you searching—it needs plenty of nutrients!

> A body that is overweight
> is usually malnourished.

Your body hopes that you're going to eat a mixed salad or steamed broccoli, but as long as you don't understand the language of your body, chances are you'll eat two thick peanut butter sandwiches, out of habit. After eating them you're still not satiated. Recognize this? When I experience a restless need-to-eat-something mood, I imagine that the cells in my body are bored and freaking out because they don't have the material to work with to keep me healthy. That image helps me to eat something healthy first, before I give in to something less healthy, such as sweets. Then I usually I don't need those sweets, or at most only a little bit.

DO YOU CRAVE FANCY CHOCOLATE, OR DOES YOUR BODY NEED MAGNESIUM?

Studies show that many women are deficient in all kinds of nutrients, especially if they've been under a lot of stress. Stress eats a large amount of your nutrients. Many women are short on the mineral magnesium. It's in chocolate. This could be why so many women crave chocolate: their bodies are desperate for magnesium.

A MALNOURISHED BODY HAS NO DESIRE TO BE ACTIVE

The last thing a malnourished body will waste energy on is unnecessary movement. A malnourished body is tired and needs to pull out all the stops for all kinds of processes in the body with the limited resources it has at its disposal. Such a body is really not going to exercise for fun.

It is no wonder you don't manage to get enough physical activity or exercise when you are malnourished. It would go against the nature of your body. The only solution is to feed your body so well that it gladly wants to be active. Only then will it happen naturally, because a healthy body likes to be active, even likes it very much!

Would you prefer to roll over and snooze longer after eight hours of sleep? Do you long to hibernate for half a year at four o'clock in the afternoon? Are you regularly too tired to do the things that you'd like to? Lack of energy is the biggest complaint I hear from women. These are all signs that your body is malnourished in one way or another.

The easiest way to get energy is from your food. Let your diet do the work for you! Your body needs plenty of energy for hormone balance, and that takes large doses of vitamins, minerals, enzymes, and trace elements. These nutrients can be found only in natural food. Change to a diet that is rich in nutrients and life force, and experience the impact.

A NATURAL DIET CONTAINS LIFE FORCE

Unprocessed, real, pure food with all its vitamins, minerals, trace elements, and other invisible and partly still unknown substances— these are your energy suppliers! This diet contains something else. I call this light, life force, or simply energy. Your diet literally contains energy that you can consume by eating. Daylight gives life energy. That's why in the spring and summer you often feel livelier and better than in the fall and winter. In spring and summer, you're outside more often and are more physically active. It's not for nothing that depressive symptoms are combated with light therapy. How do you arrange for a large dose of this life force throughout the year, so that you jump out of bed every day with great pleasure, ready to get started instead of hitting the snooze button on your alarm clock six times? Plants turn sunlight into edible light through a process known as photosynthesis. You can think of the chlorophyll in green leaves as edible sunlight. If you want more energy and life force, start by increasing the amount of green on your plate.

HOW DO YOU FEED YOUR CELLS?

The most nourishing food that you can give yourself is a big glass of fresh, organic vegetable and fruit juice from a slow juicer. By "fresh" I mean juice that you drink within 15 minutes of its being pressed. This juice contains plenty of life force. You'll find that you can't drink more than that one large glass. Your body gives the signal that it's full, because all your cells are packed with food and light. There really isn't room for more. Your stomach will soon be empty, but all the cells in your body are full. Once you've experienced this feeling, you'll never look at food the same way. You really need a slow juicer to experience this; a normal juicer destroys the life force of the food.

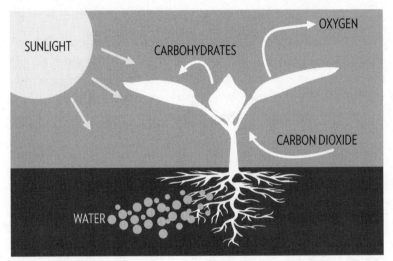

PHOTOSYNTHESIS

Seeds and sprouts pack a punch of life force. If you put a raw almond or sunflower seed in the ground, it will become a plant. If you put a roasted almond (despite how tasty it is) in the ground, nothing happens. That's what I mean by "life force." All plant foods, particularly vegetables, fruits, sprouts, herbs, seeds, kernels, and nuts, contains plenty of life force. Every day, eat some of this raw—the fresher the better—to preserve the life force. (Heating the plant above 40° Celsius, 105° Fahrenheit, destroys part of the life force.)

Let raw nuts and seeds soak overnight in water before using them. The moisture will release the life force that's inside. If you keep them moist for a few days, the start of a new plant will appear. Food that contains a lot of energy fills not only your stomach but also your cells. You're going to feel the difference from the moment you hear your alarm clock…

....

If you want more health and energy,
eat food that contains a lot of energy.

....

Processed Food Contains No Life Force

Factory foods contain absolutely no life force. They can fill your stomach, but they don't nourish your cells. Aside from all the chemical additives, that food is probably frozen, thawed, heated, pasteurized, homogenized, processed, packaged, transported, stored, and transported again, and it might be heated again before it ends up on your plate.

....

You won't know what healthy
food can do for you until you've
experienced it for yourself.

....

Organic Products Contain More Food Energy

Wild plants and food that can develop as naturally as possible contain the highest amounts of biophotons. Hence, organic agriculture gets the highest score for nutrition. Look for your country's official organic certification. Choose organic products from your own environment and eat with the seasons so that the products are as fresh as possible. Meat from animals that live outside and eat natural food is a lot healthier for you than that from the meat industry partly because of the life force that the animals have consumed. The same is true for the eggs of free-range chickens.

Eat as Nature Intended

If you eat a wide variety of food—real food, as nature intended it to be—then you'll be well on your way to good health. But I can imagine that you have many questions left, and as a former sugar junkie myself, I realize that all this is easier said than done. In Part 2 of this book I will answer a lot of your questions.

USE YOUR MICROWAVE AS A KITCHEN CUPBOARD

The microwave oven has been the subject of much debate for years. The microwave uses radio waves to agitate the water molecules in food until they begin to vibrate at the atomic level and heat is generated in the cell nucleus. Many studies show that microwaves change the DNA of our food, which our body then does not recognize as food but sees as an enemy that it must get rid of, either through excretion or by storage in our fat tissue. The original vitality of the food is destroyed in any case, and microwaving could even create cancer-causing free radicals. Please err on the side of caution: put your microwave away or pull the plug out and use it as a kitchen cupboard.

REMEMBER THIS

· For centuries people became ill and died due to a shortage of certain nutrients; it's no different now.
· Nutrition is information for all your cells. Give your body the information it needs to keep you healthy.
· Your cells require raw, pure nutrition as nature gives it to us.
· A body that suffers a nutrient deficiency will continue whining for nutrients.
· You can literally eat more energy from a food that contains more life force.

ANTI-BURNOUT SUPER JUICE

I believe that acquiring a slow juicer, with which I could make myself fresh juices, was the turning point in my burnout. There's no other way you can get so many healthy nutrients in so few gulps! If you don't have a slow juicer yet, start saving, because it will help preserve nutritional value and life force.

There are countless delicious juice recipes. I, unfortunately, have room for only one in this book. You get my favorite one, which I always choose if I feel I need something extra. Thanks to the sweetness of the beet and carrots, this recipe needs only a little fruit. This is enough for two glasses.

Here's What You Need
1 red beet
2 celery stalks
3 carrots
1 apple
a piece of ginger, about ½ inch long

Here's How You Make It
Wash the fruit and vegetables well and chop them into smaller pieces. Put everything, including the ginger, through your juicer. Pour the juice into a large glass and drink it slowly, giving it your full attention. Visualize how all your billions of body cells now are fed with the very thing they need. You can use the pulp later to bake some fine veggie burgers.

4

A MOMENT ON THE LIPS, FOREVER ON THE HIPS?

W E HAVE ALL learned that weight loss is about two simple things: eating less and exercising more. Aside from not being easy to do, it's also simply not true. Believe me: not every ounce you gain arrives by mouth! The workings of your female body are far more complex than that. There are many reasons why your body decides to store fat—not to spite you, but to protect you.

Once you know that losing weight isn't all about eating less and exercising more, you'll have meaningful knowledge you can use to achieve a healthier, slimmer body. If you're struggling with weight, it's not because your body is leaving you in the lurch. Once you understand what's happening in your body, you have the important information you need to make different choices—first to be healthy, and then to lose weight. A healthy weight is the bonus that you get with a healthy body.

PLEASE STOP COUNTING CALORIES

The biggest load of nonsense we all have come to believe is that there's a relationship between eating a certain number of calories and your weight. First, adding up calories is all pointless, because one calorie is not like the other. Second, your weight is determined by so many other factors than the number of calories you eat.

....

Lose weight to be healthy?
It works the other way around: you have
to be healthy to lose weight.

....

FEWER CALORIES BUT MORE OBESE?

The UK National Food Survey recently found that over the previous 10 years, 25 percent fewer calories had been eaten there than in the 1970s. Still, obesity in the UK increased sixfold in this same period.

All Women Are the Same, Right?

Women are advised to eat about 2,000 calories per day. For convenience, we are all lumped together, whether we're 4 foot 11 or 6 feet tall, and whether we exercise a lot or not at all. That is all wrong to start with, but that aside, if you want to lose weight, then you, as a woman, need to eat *less* than those 2,000 calories. We're told that about 1,200 to 1,500 calories a day would be suitable for weight loss. But do you think you'll lose weight if you eat 1,200 calories per day in chips and cookies for a week? And aside from your weight, how do you think you would feel, or your skin would look?

Steak or Chocolate? Same Points

This example may seem extreme, but until recently the points system at Weight Watchers (a publicly traded company with 25,000 employees worldwide!) did not differentiate between eating a steak and having a few chocolate bars—they both were worth the same number of points. Nowadays, the steak costs you fewer points, because even Weight Watchers is starting to get it: one calorie is not the same as another.

An Egg Has the Same Effect on Your Body as a Pancake, Right?

A boiled egg and a pancake contain about the same number of calories, but they affect your body in completely different ways, and that is what matters. Where you get your calories from makes a world of difference. Nutrition is information for your cells, remember? A soft-boiled egg tells your body a totally different story than a pancake.

What matters is where the calorie comes from and whether this food contributes to your health or not. A healthy weight is the result of a healthy body, one in which your hormones and organs can do their job well. No other form of healthy weight loss exists.

Dieting means fighting against your body's survival mechanism. Billions are spent on diet-industry products, which have a failure rate of 98 percent. Any other industry would long since have gone bankrupt with such dramatically bad results for their products or services. Even when people do lose weight through dieting, after a year 98 percent gain back their old weight or are even heavier. How much pain, sorrow, and frustration is involved in this outcome? There are many bizarre diets in circulation: high-protein, low-fat, low-carbohydrate, calorie-restricted, blood-type diet, seven-color diet, eat-a-lot-of-fish diet... you name it. Most diets are downright unhealthy, and for most women they don't work, because they don't tackle the hormonal cause of the weight gain. They come down to waging war against your body instead of working with your body and your hormones. Your hormones and organs decide what your body does with the nutrition. Dieting fights your survival mechanism, and you will never win that fight.

....

How could we ever have believed that it doesn't matter what type of calories you consume?

....

WHAT HAPPENS IN YOUR BODY ON A DIET?

The theory of dieting is generally that it works by consuming less food. You count calories, remove or reduce certain foods, and replace part of your diet with powders, pills, or shakes. Then what happens in your body?

As your body gets less nutrition, it will need to get its energy from somewhere else. Your essential body functions such as heart rate, digestion, and breathing will continue, and that takes energy. You would probably also like your brain to continue to work at full speed. If your body can't extract this energy from your food, the next source is your stock of glycogen.

Glycogen is the excess glucose that your body has stored in the cells of your liver and muscles so that you can quickly access this extra energy. Elite athletes often tap into this stock. Dieters do too. However, your body has also stored four grams of fluid for every gram of glycogen, so if you use the stock of glycogen, some of your body fluids will also disappear. The first few pounds you lose contain not an ounce of fat, unfortunately, but only your emergency supply of glycogen and moisture.

The next source of energy that your body turns to is the proteins in your muscles. These proteins can also be quickly converted to energy. For your body, muscles are of secondary importance for your survival, so your body will "eat" some of your muscle. Many women complain that after a few crash diets, they seem to be relatively shapeless. They're right: muscles give shape to your body. Meanwhile, some fat has also been burned, but muscles burn a lot of energy even when you're at rest. The more muscle you have, the easier it is to maintain your ideal weight or to lose weight. And speaking of calories, a couple of pounds of muscle burns hundreds of calories a day.

Women are, therefore, at a disadvantage when it comes to losing weight: it is much harder for women to build muscle. Men have more muscle; women have more fat.

Maybe now you're thinking, *Okay, those first few pounds don't count for much, plus I have to maintain my muscles, so strength training is important. But at some point, if I stick to my diet surely my body will burn fat and I'll lose weight?* Strength training is certainly a good idea, whether you want to lose weight or not. But there's a snag, and that's where so many women go wrong.

....

Diets tend to do women more harm than good,
because they never deal with the hormonal causes
and they create hormonal chaos in your body.

....

For centuries, people have had to survive in times of great food shortages. We are still built for scarcity. Your body can handle scarcity much better than abundance! From the time you go on a diet, your body will deal ever more efficiently with this limited nutrition, because it tries to keep you alive at all costs. Your body knows exactly how to do that. It will use the energy that it gets sparingly and efficiently. Your thyroid can even slow your metabolic rate to keep you going. Your body goes into survival mode. This means you lose less and less weight even while you eat very little. If you begin to eat even less than that, the weight loss will be even slower because your body will use *that* fuel very efficiently too. In the meantime, it will get harder and harder to stick to your diet, because you're going to feel more tired, dispirited, angry, or even depressed. Your body, including your brain, is longing for some nutrition, and since you're still living in a land of convenience and junk food, the risk is high that you'll end up giving in to the temptation of that pastry. Or ten pastries. Eating less if you want to lose weight permanently is not the right solution. But then, what is?

TEN REASONS YOU DON'T
LOSE WEIGHT DESPITE EATING LESS

Fat retention is a decision that your body makes, and there can be many reasons why your body does this. This is especially true for women. Women over 40 in particular know the phenomenon of "getting fat from the air": you eat and exercise exactly as you have done for years and suddenly pack on the pounds anyway! Is there anything more frustrating than the sincere feeling that the oxygen you breathe is making you fat? Believe me, I've experienced this nasty event. If you're not careful, you lose confidence in your body right when you so desperately need it, because being overweight is a sign that something is not quite right in your body and your hormones are out of balance. Let me give you ten reasons why your female body can decide not to lose weight, despite eating less and exercising more.

BE CAREFUL WITH LOW-CARB DIETS

Low-carbohydrate diets are very popular: you may eat plenty of fats and proteins as long as you don't eat carbs. This is pretty easy to maintain, and for a while you also lose weight. However, due to lack of carbohydrates (and other valuable nutrients found in healthy carbohydrates, such as B vitamins), chances are your thyroid is going to slow down. Your thyroid needs a certain amount of carbohydrates. An underactive thyroid slows your metabolism, making it more and more difficult to lose weight. Sooner or later, any one-sided diet will turn against you.

Ten Reasons

- Your intestinal flora isn't healthy and doesn't work as it should: bad bacteria have gained the upper hand. A certain configuration of bacteria in your intestinal flora can cause stubborn excess weight. Sugars in particular feed this fattening intestinal flora.
- Your thyroid decides to slow down because your adrenal glands are overloaded by stress. As a result, your metabolism slows down and you gain weight more easily.
- Your adrenal glands produce lots of cortisol because you've been under too much stress for a long time. Stress disrupts, among other things, your hormone balance, which makes you store fat instead of burning it. Stress can make you fat.
- Your body continuously produces too much insulin because your cells have become insensitive to insulin. With insulin in your blood, it is impossible to burn fat.
- Your liver has trouble detoxifying and disposing of hormone-disrupting substances, including xenoestrogens. Your fat cells decide to store these substances because otherwise they can harm your body. Your body stores them in your fat cells. The more xenoestrogens, the more fat cells.
- As you get older, your muscle mass slowly diminishes, making your metabolism slow down. The less muscle you have, the lower your metabolism and the more difficult it is to lose weight.
- Your metabolism is confused because of years of (crash) diets, and is constantly in survival mode. It no longer trusts that there will always be enough food and stores everything you eat directly as fat.
- Your body lacks some important nutrients it needs to be able to burn fat, such as magnesium, zinc, or the B vitamins.
- You use medications with side effects that cause weight gain and/or make it difficult to lose weight. Please note that the contraceptive pill is also a drug.
- Your metabolism slows down in the end anyway because you get older, even though you do strength training and look after your muscles.

The effect of each and every one of these ten causes—in which, as you can see, not one single calorie is mentioned—may be that you can't lose weight or even that you get fatter while you eat less. There are many other causes: a viral infection, intestinal inflammation, or Lyme disease, for example.

Persistent obesity is a call for help from your body. If you provide for hormone balance, healthy intestinal flora, and healthy adrenal and thyroid glands, if you support your liver in detoxifying, keep your muscles in good shape, and don't overload your body with too many polluting substances or an overdose of stress, you will help your body to get back in balance and achieve a healthy weight. This is a lot, it's true, but you won't have to count even one calorie!

Women Lose Weight in the Kitchen, Not at the Gym

If you do decide to spend more good time in the kitchen, chances are you'll lose weight. With healthy food, your hormones and organs will become balanced, and a healthy weight will generally follow as a bonus. Be patient, and be aware that a healthy weight is not the same size for every woman. The bottom line is that you'll have a body that feels right to you and that is full of energy.

Physical activity and sports are very healthy, but unfortunately, we women lose less weight this way than men. Even at rest, muscle cells consume more energy than fat cells. If you have a lot of muscle, your metabolism is more active and you'll lose weight more easily. Muscles are fine partners in the fight against obesity. But exercising does little for your weight, especially if your metabolism is low. Research shows that exercising makes women hungry. Less sitting and regular walking or cycling speed up your metabolism in a good way. Physical activity before breakfast, on an empty stomach, is also a great way to speed up your metabolism.

....

The secret of slim women is not diets.
The secret is that they know they *do* have
to eat and also *what* they should eat.

....

YOUR HORMONES DETERMINE WHAT YOUR BODY DOES WITH YOUR NUTRIENTS

Being overweight is a signal that your body is out of balance, even if these extra pounds are caused by you eating too much unhealthy food for a long time. Because of course, there *are* women who eat too much. Sometimes *far* too much. But even then, it's your hormones that cause you to eat too much. Not having a sense of satiety or eating because of sadness, frustration, or need for consolation is also the work of your hormones. I've never met a woman who could comfort herself with a celery stalk; for that we need something else.

Hormones determine what the body does with the nutrients it gets. Is your body using them to build muscle or for fat storage, and where is that fat then stored? Your hormones determine your appetite, and even your addictive patterns. If you can no longer stop after that first handful of peanuts or those first two cookies, it's your hormones that are making you eat like a zombie. You will become healthier and leaner precisely by eating the right things. Are you too heavy? Stop dieting and go eat—*healthy* food. Food that gives your body as many nutrients as possible, and at the same time as few polluting substances as possible.

REMEMBER THIS

- Counting calories to maintain weight is unhealthy nonsense.
- Almost all diets cause massive hormonal chaos in a woman's body and do more harm than good.
- Your hormones determine what your body does with the nutrients it gets.

- There can be many reasons why you're not losing weight despite eating less food and exercising more.
- Persistent obesity is a call for help from your body.
- A slim body is the bonus that you get with a healthy body. You get a healthy body by first eating healthy food.
- A healthy body craves physical activity.

CRUNCHY CAULIFLOWER PIZZA

I've made quite a few recipes "greener" by replacing starch with vegetables. This is my favorite pizza recipe, with a cauliflower crust. No, it absolutely does not taste like cauliflower, and yes, it really is crisp. You can load up this pizza with everything you think is delicious and healthy. A pizza without cheese is not a pizza, in my opinion—that's why I got to work with buffalo mozzarella and goat cheese. The artichoke hearts come from a glass jar for convenience.

Here's What You Need (for 3 people)

For the crust

1 medium cauliflower
2 eggs
⅞ cups of almond flour
1 cup of rolled oats (fine oat flakes)
2 tablespoons Italian seasoning
fresh pepper and Celtic Sea salt
1 tablespoon olive oil

For the topping

6 tomatoes
1 red onion
1 jar artichoke hearts (14 ounces)
4½ ounces buffalo mozzarella
1 chunk of spicy goat cheese
1 cup passata (sieved tomatoes from a bottle)
1 tablespoon Italian herbs
a handful of arugula, chopped
olive oil

Here's How You Make It

Preheat oven to 350°F. Line a rectangular baking sheet with parchment paper. Remove the cauliflower's leaves and hard stem. Chop the florets in your food processor until they look like white rice. In a small bowl, beat the eggs. In a separate, large bowl, mix the cauliflower with the almond flour, oats, Italian seasoning, fresh pepper, sea salt, and olive oil. Make a well in the center and pour the egg mixture in. Stir well with a fork. It will be more of a thick batter than a normal pizza dough. Scoop the dough onto your cookie sheet and press it with your fingers into a rectangular shape with a raised edge. The crust should be approximately ½ inch thick. Bake in the oven for about 20 minutes. The raised edges will be slightly brown.

Meanwhile, slice the tomatoes. Chop the onion and drain the artichoke hearts. Cut the mozzarella and goat cheese into slices.

Remove the crust from the oven and spread a layer of passata over it. Cover the pizza crust with the tomatoes, artichoke hearts, and cheeses. Sprinkle with the herbs. Put the pizza back in the oven for about 15 minutes. Just before serving, sprinkle generously with the chopped arugula and some olive oil.

PART TWO

The Energetic Woman's Nutrition Compass

5

THE BASIC PRINCIPLE

———————

I F YOU IMAGINE your path to vitality and health as a journey, then it's handy to have a compass on hand. It helps you reach your goal. It doesn't prescribe your destination or the speed at which you'll travel. You decide your destination, your direction, and your pace: you're at the wheel of your life. The Energetic Woman's Nutrition Compass works like a compass: it helps you set the course of your diet for a journey to more health and vitality. The Compass is guided by one basic principle—your North—and seven key points. Using this basis, you determine your route. In this part of the book, you will first read about the basic principle, and after that I'll give you the seven points.

YOUR UNIQUE PATH

———————

The question I get most from my clients is, "Marjolein, how do I sustain healthy eating habits?" I always say that there is no such thing as "sustain" when you are on a journey to learn and experience something new. Sustain is a word that fits a strict regime in which you can do only right or wrong. Traveling under the guidance of the Nutrition Compass means you cannot take a wrong turn.

See changing your diet as like learning to play an instrument. You have to practice; you won't master it in a day. At first the going will be rough and it won't sound like music. But if you practice a little every day, you'll gradually improve and become more and more skilled. Then one day you'll effortlessly play a beautiful melody and you can no longer imagine why you ever felt it was so hard. It's the same when you change your diet.

There Is No Failure

The Nutrition Compass does not give daily menus—there *are* no daily menus that are appropriate for all women. I am convinced that this is an important reason why women don't maintain a diet: they're following something that doesn't meet their personal needs. If you do that, sooner or later your body will start to protest. One deviation from the prescribed daily menu will make you feel like a failure and you could easily fall back into old unhealthy patterns. This will not happen with the Nutrition Compass. Failure does not exist if you think of learning a new diet as being like learning to play an instrument.

You might be someone who likes a strictly prescribed daily meal plan telling you exactly what and how much you should eat. I don't believe in that method, for two reasons.

First, you're unique and your body is unique. Every woman requires a different quantity and combination of foods. Maybe today you need something different from what you'll need three months from now, when you're in a stressful period of your life.

Second, I believe that every woman knows exactly what nutrition she needs, and this "knowing" is what I would like to wake up in you. There's only one person who can determine what you need, and that's you. Use your common sense and your intuition when it comes to nutrition, and learn again to listen to the signals your body sends. Only then will you find out what helps you thrive.

....

You're on your way to learn something new:
a new diet. Failure does not
exist if you're learning something new.

....

Give Yourself Time

It may be that you don't yet understand what your body is trying to tell you. Many women have lost contact with their bodies. As a client of mine once said, "I listen really, really closely to my body, Marjolein, but I hear nothing!" Allow yourself time to rebuild your relationship with your body. Here's a starting point you probably know: when you're really sick, your body tells you it's a bad idea to eat. Your body needs all its energy to recover, and at that point digestion just requires too much energy. You won't be hungry even if you haven't eaten for two days.

....

When you have cravings, you probably ask
yourself, "What do I feel like having?"
The Nutrition Compass invites you to ask
your body, "What do I need?"

....

Learn to Understand the
Language of Your Body Again

This is what I mean by listening to your body. As you eat healthier foods, you will better understand the language of your body and you'll know what you need. A healthy communication will start between you and your body. You'll find that your body is going to increasingly ask for healthy things and not for junk food or candy, or you'll know more clearly when you're thirsty, not hungry. Maybe you can't imagine this now, but I promise you that there will come a point when you will know what is good for you. Be patient with yourself: as you bring your hormones back in balance, you will reawaken the wisdom of your body.

THE BASIC PRINCIPLE: NUTRITION IN,
BULK AND CONTAMINATION OUT

The Nutrition Compass separates nutrition from bulk foods, "empty" calories, and contamination. Once you know which category a food falls into, the rest is simple: take care to eat more healthy food, and phase out the junk and contamination as much as possible.

Your body is a slow organism and needs time to adapt, so it's important to change your diet step by step. Maybe you have tried to eat healthier before but you haven't been able to stay on that path long enough. Often, we fall back into old, unhealthy eating patterns for a variety of reasons—reasons that are not always easy to avoid, such as stress, hurry, or painful emotions that want to be soothed with sweets. But people with healthy eating patterns also experience stress, lack of time, and painful emotions, yet they manage to avoid a bad diet. These reasons will keep coming, so how do you make sure they no longer get such a grip on your diet?

The Secret to Easily Changing Your Diet

I will reveal to you the secret method for easily changing your diet. The trick is to feed yourself healthy food that is delicious and simple to prepare. If you want to change your diet, focus on everything that is healthy and make sure you ingest as much of it as possible. Your body is desperate for a healthy diet and plenty of nutrients.

Most diets are based on limitations and what you should *not* eat. From day one, they have a list of what you aren't allowed. When you suddenly omit what your body is used to (and addicted to), that's stressful for your body. Willpower might help you for a while but often not very long. The Nutrition Compass starts with eating healthy things, and you will soon find that you are feeling more energetic and healthier. Only then is it easier to leave the unhealthy things behind and feel like engaging in more physical activity. Say you eat three meals and two snacks every day; that's 35 times a week. If five of those times you eat following the points of the Nutrition

Compass, that's a nice start. The next week it might be eight times. The week after that, ten.

....

It's about what you usually eat, not
what you occasionally eat.

....

Slowly the ingredients in your kitchen will change and you'll become more competent and faster at preparing them. And you're going to feel better... until at some point you'll realize it's become habit and you no longer want it any other way.

....

You don't fight malnutrition by
avoiding unhealthy foods. You combat
malnutrition by eating real food.

....

**Go Eat Real Food and Make It
as Tasty as Possible**

By "real food" I mean all-natural products that your body recognizes as nutrients and that it can use to nourish itself. The products are packed with nutrients just as nature intended them for us: vegetables, fruits, herbs, sprouts, raw nuts, seeds, tubers, seeds, eggs, meat, and fish. A simple rule: Real nutrition is basically something with just one ingredient—an apple, a piece of chicory, an egg, or a trout... that's real food. The art is to combine some of these products in your kitchen so you get something tasty without it taking a lot of time.

The good news is that you can eat quite a lot of this healthy, natural food. Ever since my adolescence, I've had to watch my weight. I've often dieted, and I felt constantly hungry. I've never eaten so much as I have over the past few years, but I eat differently. The point is to eat as many nutrients as possible. You may be surprised by how much healthy food you can eat without gaining weight. But okay... you should, of course, not overdo it.

If you are struggling with your weight, you may think, *But I may gain even more extra weight!* My experience is that this is almost never the case. Maybe at the beginning, when you can't yet feel how much food your body needs and you still eat out of habit rather than out of need, but if you really feed your body nutritious food, you'll notice that the need for food laden with chemicals or your tendency for sweets or for overeating will decrease. Your taste buds are renewed every seven days, so if you manage to avoid eating sweets for a week, you're over the worst. You'll find that healthy foods fill you up differently. It really *feels* different.

Maybe you think, *But I already mostly eat all fresh and natural food!* Then you're on the right track. But unfortunately, some natural products can be contaminated—more on this in the next chapters. And maybe you do not expect this: Enjoying a piece of homemade apple pie in the good company of a dear friend, or a glass of wine at a festive dinner party, also falls, in my opinion, under "real" nutrition. Even a piece of white bread with thick butter and chocolate-hazelnut spread is not always 100 percent bad for you … if you do it once in a while and really enjoy it!

Are You Allowed to Enjoy "Unhealthy" Food?

If you enjoy food, your body's reaction will be totally different than it will if you're thinking, with every bite, *I'm being bad—this is too much sugar. I was determined not to do this. I'm so mad at myself again!* These thoughts give your body stress. If you occasionally give in to a craving for a chocolate-hazelnut spread sandwich, enjoy that too! See it as a treat.

Phase Out Empty Calories and Junk as Much as Possible

Junk food and processed and packaged foods full of empty calories are, directly or indirectly, endocrine-disrupting chemicals. By "empty calories," I mean everything you eat that fills you up but provides little nutritional value. Think of soft drinks, cookies, candy, desserts, sweetened milk products, ice cream, chips, pretzels, and ready-made "meals," and everything that comes in packets, pouches, and boxes. Almost everything that is not made by nature falls into this category. These things will fill your stomach, often with the addictive combination of sugar, salt, and unhealthy fats, but they won't nourish your body. Furthermore, filling your stomach is not as innocent a thing to do as you may think.

Soft drinks and sweets are empty calories: calories with no nutrients. All food, however, has an effect on your body. Therefore, it's not entirely accurate to speak about "empty" calories. If you eat a piece of cake or drink a glass of cola, you consume a lot of sugar. To get these sugars out of your body again, much must be done. As soon as the food enters your body, your body determines if it can be put to good use, and if not, how it needs to be safely disposed of. For this disposal process, your body needs, among other things, B vitamins and magnesium. Your body will use up all of your stores of these nutrients to get rid of the sugars. And wouldn't you know it—B vitamins and magnesium are two nutrients you desperately need to make you feel energetic!

....

Do you pay a lot of attention to the outside of your body? Focus on the inside and what you put in it for a while. The impact this has on the outside will surprise you.

....

You've probably felt lethargic or even exhausted after an afternoon break with lots of sweets or a pancake with syrup and a glass of cola. You now know why: your body is working hard to get sugars safely back out of your body.

Pollutants Disrupt Hormones

By "pollutants" I mean all the toxic substances that may impair your health if you ingest a lot of them. Many factory food products contain toxic substances. Polluters include a large number of permitted additives—preservatives and colors and flavors, the material on the inside of plastic bottles, cans, and packages, the chemical sweeteners in "light" products, the chemical (trans) fats in margarine and other vegetable oil products, and the acrylamide found in all deep-fried food. Also, the pesticides on nonorganic fruits and vegetables fall under toxic substances. Nonorganic meat and dairy can be contaminated with antibiotics, growth hormones, and vaccines. Wild fish can be contaminated with heavy metals such as mercury, and farmed fish with antibiotics and growth hormones. I know, it's not nice to realize this, but for your health's sake it's important to be aware of it. I don't want to scare you, though. Just be discerning about what you put into your body.

What's Okay from Food Factories?

Not everything that comes from a factory is junk or empty food or contaminated. Think of a packet of butter, fast-frozen vegetables and fruits, herbs, healthy fats and oils, raw nuts, beans in glass jars, and so on. Fresh is always better, but because you also, of course, like convenience, these products are a welcome addition to fresh, natural products. I use them as well. At the end of this book (Appendix A) is a table in which I indicate which products you can use and which you are wiser to avoid.

Empty calories don't exist. Every calorie has some effect on your body.

THE SEVEN POINTS OF THE NUTRITION COMPASS

As well as its basic principle, the Nutrition Compass has seven points to help you to stay on a healthy path.

The first three points elaborate on the first part of the basic principle: get healthy food into your body; start with food that's good for your hormones.

· Eat and drink as nature provided.
· Do not be afraid of healthy fats (and eat them!).
· Eat plenty of plants.

Points 4, 5, and 6 elaborate on the second part: get empty calories and junk food and contamination out of your diet; after that, begin to avoid less healthy food that disrupts your hormones.

· Be smarter than candy.
· Cow's milk is for calves.
· Intestines do not like gluten.

Point 7 emphasizes the importance of variety, including the use of supplements.

· Eat a wide variety of foods (but don't eat too much).

REMEMBER THIS

· Changing your diet is like learning to play an instrument: do it step by step and be patient with yourself.
· No prescribed daily menu is suitable for all women; every woman's body is unique.
· Start with eating healthy food. Then focus on phasing out anything less healthy.
· Don't be too strict; if you eat something that's not so healthy, really allow yourself to enjoy it.

QUICK BLUEBERRY JAM WITH CHIA SEEDS

Chia seeds are one of my favorite superfoods; they contain complete proteins and omega-3 fatty acids, and a variety of minerals. You can easily make a pudding or jam with them. I grind them finely, just like flax seeds, in small amounts in a coffee grinder and store them in the refrigerator, but you can also use them whole. The blue color of blueberries comes from anthocyanin, a substance that has many health benefits.

Here's What You Need
¾ cup blueberries (tightly packed)
1 tablespoon lemon juice
1 teaspoon maple syrup
½ teaspoon vanilla extract
¾ tablespoon chia seed

Here's How You Make It
Put all the ingredients except the chia seeds in a small saucepan and heat slowly. With a wooden spoon, mash the blueberries as they soften. Stir until it looks like jam. Then add the chia seeds and remove the pan from the heat. Let stand for 5 minutes. Put in sterilized canning jars. Store the jam in the refrigerator. It lasts only a week, so keep it in sight and don't forget that you've made it.

6

POINT 1:
EAT AND DRINK AS
NATURE PROVIDES

———————

I F 80 PERCENT OF your diet comes from a wide variety of foods made as nature intended—real food, in other words—then you're already doing very well. You're giving your body and your hormones the information they need to keep you healthy and vital. If you then eat something not so healthy, your body will dispose of it without any problem.

EAT WITH THE SEASONS

Products from nature usually spoil quickly. The fresher the better, because some of the nutrients are lost between harvesting and the supermarket. There's little we can do about this. If you like bananas and live in a nontropical climate, you'll have to accept the travel time because bananas don't grow well outside the tropics. Of course, you can strive for freshness when it comes to local products. As much as possible, eat with the seasons. If you eat the freshest fruits and vegetables, they'll also be the cheapest.

TIP: Hang a chart showing when local foods are in season on the inside of a kitchen cabinet door, so you always know what foods on offer are fresh. You can find charts from many agricultural agencies.

ORGANIC REALLY DOES MAKE SENSE

Nature gives us products without pesticides, and that's for a good reason. In Chapter 2 you read how toxic substances may be hormone disruptors and how they disrupt your endocrine system. These hormone disruptors are all around us—we can never completely avoid them. We can, however, as much as possible, choose organic products. Organic farming goes a step further when it comes to healthy soil management, environmental care, and nutritional value. These products are for sale under official national organic marks. True, organic products are more expensive, but that has a reason. Admittedly, with the naked eye we see little difference between an organic and nonorganic broccoli. However, you get three birds with one stone:

1. Organic broccoli contains more healthy substances than nonorganic broccoli. These plants haven't been sprayed with chemical pesticides; they make substances to protect themselves from their enemies, such as fungi and caterpillars. These substances, phytonutrients, also protect against all kinds of illnesses, including cancer. It's important to eat as much of these substances as possible. If a plant is sprayed, it makes less or none of these substances: the pesticide dispels the fungus or caterpillars, so the plant no longer needs to do it for itself.

2. Pesticides contain hormone disruptors and slowly poison your body. If your liver is not able to dispose of them, xenoestrogens accumulate. This results in a disruption of your hormone balance, leading to estrogen dominance and overweight.

3. There is some discussion about whether organic products contain more vitamins and minerals than nonorganic products.

Organic plant products have been grown in better-quality soil, from which they have been able to absorb vitamins and minerals. Organic animal products come from animals that have been able to eat natural foods in more space and that are treated better than factory-farmed animals. Which foods do you think would contain more nutrients?

Organic makes sense, but do what is possible for you. Not everything I eat is always organic because sometimes the price difference is too big, and eating at a restaurant usually means not eating organic.

Online, you'll find annual "Dirty Dozen" lists of the fruits and vegetables with the most pesticide residue. You can see at a glance which fruits and vegetables are most contaminated and thus which ones you'd be better to buy organic. Always wash nonorganic products well, preferably in a bowl of water with a dash of vinegar.

YOUR BODY RECOGNIZES THE DIFFERENCE

Nutrition is more than just the sum of vitamins and minerals. A plant that grows in artificial light with measured amounts of fertilizer is a different plant from one that has been in the open air and had to work hard for food. A chicken that has been allowed to scurry outside is a different animal from a battery chicken fed on soy that has been stressed her whole life. Even if you don't see it, your body recognizes the difference.

USE LOTS OF AGES IF YOU WANT LOTS OF WRINKLES

AGE stands for advanced glycation end product. It's a difficult term to indicate a bonding between sugars and proteins from your diet. The resulting compounds provide your body with a lot of free radicals.

Free radicals are molecules with an aggressive streak. This aggression leads them to pull apart molecular structures, breaking down your cells and even damaging your DNA. Damaged cells lead to accelerated cellular aging, wrinkles, and, if many cells are corrupted, illness. All kinds of joint problems, high blood pressure, arteriosclerosis, cardiovascular disease, kidney problems, brain diseases, eye problems, diabetes, and obesity can be a result of too many AGEs in your body.

AGEs arise naturally in your body due to normal metabolism; these AGEs are unavoidable. Foods like meat, fish, dairy, and nuts are rich in AGEs. Here you can start making choices. But the most damaging AGEs are created by the processing of food in manufacturing plants. Pasteurization, sterilization, and refining increase the AGEs in food, as does heat. Many factory foods have already been heated once, before they even get to your kitchen. All chemical substances added in the manufacturing process to enhance fragrance, color, flavor, mouth feel, and shelf life result in more AGEs.

Unfortunately, our noses and our taste buds find certain AGEs very delicious. Something baking, grilling, frying, roasting, deepfrying, caramelizing, or cooking au gratin—delicious, right? Unfortunately, the higher the temperature and the longer the food is modified, the more AGEs are in it.

You Can Drastically Reduce AGEs in Your Diet

· Avoid factory-processed foods as much as possible.
· Warm your natural foods at low temperatures. Steaming, poaching, or cooking for a short time is fine.
· Learn about delicious raw food cooking and enjoy "raw" treats with your coffee or tea, such as the avocado-lemon tarts in this book, instead of having the usual (homemade) cookies or cake.

· View all food that has been heated to a high temperature as a treat. Enjoy it but don't eat too much of it.

KEEP HEALTHY FOOD HEALTHY

Nature gives us a great range of healthy products. The most life force is in raw food. It's smart, therefore, to keep part of your diet unprocessed and eat raw. I recommend that you eat half your vegetables raw. Eat a mixed salad as lunch and/or at dinner daily and you're already there.

Warming Is Healthier Than Heating

If you want to heat your food, it's better to use low temperatures for a short period to scald, steam, or poach. In this way you retain nutrients as much as possible. Cooking at high temperatures removes a large part of the nutrients and the life force. In addition, the food is then full of AGES.

> Heating may make food
> very tasty, but this doesn't mean
> that it's very good for you.

AGEs Inhibit Leptin

Leptin is the hormone that lets you say, at the right time, "I've eaten enough." If you already don't have enough of this hormone, then you have another reason to avoid AGEs as much as possible, because they inhibit the action of leptin. You can devour a bowl of roasted nuts in a few minutes; a bowl of raw nuts, however, fills you up quite quickly. That difference arises because roasted nuts have an inhibiting effect on leptin.

Avoid Food Packaged in Plastic, Cardboard, Tin, and Aluminum

Many factory food products are packaged in plastic. Depending on the type of plastic, it can contain hormone-disrupting substances. Especially with fluids and fats packaged in plastic, there's a risk of contamination with xenoestrogens; these leak into the food from the packaging.

DO YOU KNOW THE RECYCLING CODE?

Plastic must be marked with a recycling code. This code, a number from 1 to 7, is often between three arrows at the bottom of the product. It tells you about the type of plastic. Avoid, as much as possible, code 1 (PET, or nylon), code 3 (PVC, usually not found in food packaging), and code 7 (other varieties). Code 7 is a collection of everything that is not under 1 to 6. Your particular plastic may be innocent, but the harmful BPA (bisphenol A) is also under code 7.

BPA is a harmful xenoestrogen found especially in the plastic layer on the inside of cans and cardboard packaging. From this plastic covering it leaks into food. Intake of BPA is associated with polycystic ovary syndrome (PCOS), liver problems, cardiovascular diseases, diabetes, and immune system problems. In a Harvard School of Public Health study, the blood of subjects who had eaten canned soup for five days showed 20 times more BPA than was found in the blood of subjects who had eaten freshly made soup.

Try not to buy food in plastic bottles, cardboard packaging, tin, or aluminum; it can contain hormone-disrupting substances. Glass is excellent packaging material. At home, try to store food in glass, earthenware, or BPA-free plastic. If you need to carry water, buy water bottles made of glass, stainless steel or BPA-free plastic.

WHAT IS NUTRITION WHEN IT COMES FROM A FOOD FACTORY?

Processed food marketing goes out of its way to give the impression that a manufacturing facility works the same as our kitchen but on a very large scale. From advertising and packaging, we get the impression that they use only the freshest ingredients and prepare the food just as we would at home. To make it easy for us, they have bought, cleaned, and tastily cooked fresh products, and the only thing we need to do is to warm it up and maybe to add a few extra things we like to eat... as if the manufacturer were a caring neighbor who has cooked for us during a period when we ourselves were busy. This couldn't be further from the truth.

Don't Look Only at Additives

A food processing facility nowadays seems more like a paint factory than like your neighbor's kitchen. In her book *Swallow This*, investigative journalist Joanna Blythman describes her undercover visit to the annual fair called Food Ingredients Europe, a mega trade show for suppliers and buyers of the ingredients used by the modern food industry. Throughout the whole exhibition she found hardly anything that reminded her of food. The food industry turned out to be the domain of scientists and engineers. The trade show was about anti-foaming agents, emulsifying agents, foam formers, solvents for flavorings, glazing agents, emulsifying salts, propellants, flour treatment agents, flavors, binders, and many other raw materials. What was traded was not ingredients like apples and onions but acesulfame K, azodicarbonamide, ammonium chloride, tertiary butylhydroquinone (TBHQ), phosphoric acid, monosodium glutamate, antifreeze, and ethylenediaminetetraacetic acid.

The companies trying to sell their products to the food industry turned out to be the same companies that supply producers of animal feed, cosmetics, detergents, cleaning products, building materials, plastics, adhesive fabrics, paper, and industrial chemicals. Chemical companies such as Omya, Corbion, Helm AG, and DKSH also turned out to be the suppliers of the modern food industry. Blythman writes, "They experience no cognitive dissonance in providing components not only for your ready meals, but also for your fly spray, air freshener, shower sealant, deodorant, computer casing, scratch-resistant car coating, paint and glue."[1] Do you understand now why I call factory food fake food?

The Food Industry's "Clean Labels"

We don't see these names of chemical ingredients and flavor enhancers on food product labels because the food industry knows very well that if we consumers knew what is in their products, we would no longer buy them. Instead they work ever harder on "clean labels." Monosodium glutamate, or, in Europe, the E number E621, is replaced by the innocent-sounding "yeast extract," and butylated hydroxyanisole (E320) by "extract of rosemary"; however, E320 doesn't resemble the eponymous herb at all but is an extraction of chemical solvents such as hexane, ethanol, and acetone.

In the last few years, in Europe, anyone who wants to eat healthy has learned to pay attention to the E numbers on the packaging. But Blythman notes that paying attention to additives on labels is no longer enough. Because of "clean labels," we need to be smarter than that. The healthiest solution seems to be avoiding packaged and processed commercial food whenever you can. This is the only way to avoid chemical substances, and thus possible hormone disruptors.

So use fresh products as much as possible. You will soon notice how wonderful your food tastes if you no longer allow food-industry "flavor bursts" in your mouth.

....

Cooking with scissors (to cut open the packaging)
always comes at the expense of your
hormone balance and therefore your health.

....

How Does the Food Industry Keep You Eating?

There's another good reason to avoid factory food as much as possible. Every company in the food industry is fighting for a piece of your stomach and mine. It's a thorn in their side that our stomachs aren't larger, because they want to sell us as much as possible. This gets easier if we become addicted to their products. More and more research indicates that, in particular, food that contains a combination of sugars, fats, and a little salt is as addictive as cocaine, morphine, and nicotine. It triggers your brain to make dopamine, the feel-good hormone. In prehistoric times, people often had to struggle to find enough food to survive. Along with a filled stomach, dopamine was a reward for finding and eating energy-rich food.

FOOD ADDICTION: AN UNDERESTIMATED PHENOMENON

We're especially fond of sugar, but you'll never just empty your sugar bowl during a binge. You would tire of only sugar quickly enough. Yet we eat and drink too much sugar packaged in soft drinks, cookies, cakes, chocolate, ice cream, and sandwich spreads, as well as chips, pretzels, pizza, and other savory snacks. All are combinations of sugars, fats, and salt. Sure, there's salt in vanilla ice cream and sugar in chips, and that's for a reason. But most of these products are sweetened with fructose, which disrupts your satiation hormone leptin. By eating them you lose your ability to feel full at the right time and you get a dopamine surge like you would with cocaine. Is it any wonder that so many people are addicted to food and struggling with their weight?

NATURE KNOWS NO PRODUCTS WITH SUGARS, FAT, AND SALT

We live in a world in which addictive foods containing a mix of plenty of fats, sugars, and salt are available every day. However, nowhere in nature are these three ingredients found in one product. Probably to our advantage: there's a good chance that our ancestors would have sat like junkies under the trees with fruits like these, and humanity would have become extinct long ago.

RATS BECOME ADDICTED TO SUGARS IN SUPERMARKET FOOD

Scientists at the Princeton Neuroscience Institute found out that sugar-conditioned rats that suddenly got no sugar exhibited withdrawal symptoms similar to those of drug users, such as retreat to a safe tunnel and teeth chattering. They were too frightened to explore as they normally would. Once they had access to sugars again, they overate even more, and they started drinking more alcohol as well. They had become real junkies.[2]

....

You are what you eat. If you don't know what you eat, how can you know who you are?

....

The Food Industry Is Looking for Your "Seventh Heaven" Feeling

In his book *Salt Sugar Fat: How the Food Giants Hooked Us,* investigative journalist Michael Moss describes the quest of the food industry to find our "seventh heaven" feeling. That is the point at which we get the greatest dopamine surge (and thus can become the most addicted) in combination with the point at which we still find the product tasty. Too much sugar, fat, and salt can in fact yield a higher dopamine surge but may also ensure that a product doesn't taste good anymore or that we've had enough of it after a few bites.

Moss writes, "Some of the largest companies are now using brain scans to examine how we react neurologically to certain foods, especially to sugar. … The world's biggest ice cream maker, Unilever, for instance, parlayed its brain research into a brilliant marketing campaign that sells the eating of ice cream as a 'scientifically proven' way to make ourselves happy."[3] In his book, Moss explains that this is not normal sugar, salt, and fat, like you use in the kitchen:

> I would find out that one of the most fascinating, and unsettling, aspects of the role of salt, sugar, and fat in processed foods is the way the industry, in an effort to boost their operation, has sought to alter their physical shape and structure. Scientists at Nestlé are currently fiddling with the distribution and shape of fat globules to affect their absorption rate and, as it's known in the industry, "mouth feel." At Cargill, the world's leading supplier of salt, scientists are altering the physical shape of salt by pulverizing it into a fine powder to hit the taste buds faster and harder, improving what the company calls its "flavor burst." Sugar is being altered in myriad ways as well. The sweetest component of simple sugar, fructose, has been crystallized into an additive that increases the attractiveness of foods. Scientists have also designed stimulants that boosts the sweetness of sugar to two hundred times its natural strength.[4]

Large food companies have hundreds of millions of dollars available for research. They do brain research, among other things, to make us eat as much of their products as possible. Their products are highly addictive. This fight is unfair.

....

The food industry can create food that
makes you hungry as you eat it.

....

Be the Boss of Your Stomach

The food industry has succeeded in stretching and thereby enlarg-
ing our stomachs. The number of stomach reduction surgeries has
ballooned over the last 15 years. In 2013, 10,000 people in the Netherlands alone had a gastric bypass, an operation that is not without
risks. Twenty percent of public hospitals in the Netherlands perform
this operation; the number of private clinics that provide gastric
bands and gastric bypasses increases every year. But if you eat pure
foods given to us as nature intended, you'll never need a gastric band.
Your body will automatically tell you when enough is enough. Then
you won't need to have any willpower at all.

CLEAN DRINKING WATER:
THE PRIMARY MEDICINE

You are composed of 75 percent water. Water is the basis of your
vitality and health, and it is wise to think about it as a necessary ele-
ment of your daily menu. If you drink enough water, everything in
your body will run smoother and faster, because water thins your
blood. Nutrients will reach the cells that need them more quickly,
and waste materials will be more easily excreted. Your brain will get
more oxygen because oxygen is transported through your blood.

If your body is drying out, you won't feel very energetic. Prolonged dehydration is the basis of many health problems. As you
get older, it is even more important to ensure adequate hydration.
A deficiency of fluids in your body can lead to all sorts of physical
and mental complaints. With aging, it seems to be more difficult to
experience thirst. One study shows that even after 24 hours without
water, elderly subjects still didn't feel thirsty.

As you get older, your skin loses capacity for adequate moisture retention. If you also *deprive* it of moisture, it will age even faster. So drink plenty of water to prevent all those emerging wrinkles!

Aim for Eight Glasses a Day

Try to drink about eight glasses (two liters) of water every day. Water, that is—so no soft drinks, fruit juices, flavored water, coffee, or black tea. You can partly replace water with herbal tea, but vary the types of tea: each herb has its own effect on your body. Try not to drink while eating, because that disturbs your digestion. Also, no drinking ice-cold water: your body needs water at body temperature or preferably room temperature; otherwise, it's a cold shock for your body, and it takes energy to warm your core back up.

HOW DO YOU DRINK EIGHT GLASSES OF WATER A DAY?

The easiest way to drink this much water is to set a timer on your cellphone for 11:00 a.m., 4:00 p.m., and 8:00 p.m. Drink two large glasses of water at each of these times plus two glasses immediately after getting up in the morning. The latter is very healthy for jump-starting your digestive system and replacing the fluids you've lost during the night.

The Quality of Our Drinking Water

The Netherlands is considered a country with high-quality drinking water, and perhaps where you live is too. Yet there are some disadvantages even in places like ours, because our drinking water is no longer as nature intended it. Unfortunately, it contains undesirable substances such as chlorine, lime, copper, lead, and the remnants of antibiotics, pesticides, and, increasingly, medications.

Where I live, our drinking water is extracted from surface water and groundwater. But research shows that the quality of these sources often no longer meets standards because they're polluted with chemicals, and only 60 out of about 10,000 of these are controlled for before the water reaches us, the customer.[5] The quality of our drinking water is determined only on the basis of the controlled substances. What about all the other chemicals?

More and more tap-water filter systems are on the market to filter out unwanted substances. Some good systems filter out 99 percent of the drug residue. Water filters not only remove pollutants from the water, but also vitalize the water, which means better absorption for your body. In some cases, they even add minerals. In addition to being a lot healthier for you, filtered water also tastes better.

....

Do you find it difficult to drink only
tap water because you don't like it? Filtered
tap water is not only tastier but also
easier for your body to absorb.

....

The question is: Is your drinking water good enough for you? If you drink enough water and you feel excellent, unburdened by symptoms or inconveniences (persistent obesity counts as an inconvenience), then apparently your body is disposing of the concentrations of chemicals well. However, if you have symptoms or diseases, save up for a good filter system that also removes medication residues from your drinking water.

REMEMBER THIS

· Examine everything you eat or drink to see if it still looks like the product nature created for us.

- As much as possible, eat organic.
- Limit the heating of food at high temperatures.
- Please be aware that everything from food factories has been highly processed, and has often been designed to make you eat as much of it as possible.
- Consider water an important part of your daily diet. Consider filtering your drinking water to remove hormone disruptors.

STUFFED CARROT SALAD
WITH TAHINI DRESSING

No, we're not going to hollow out a carrot and fill it. What I want to show you is that a healthy, energetic salad does not consist of watery iceberg lettuce, tomato, and cucumber slices; that kind of salad will only make you hungry and leave you feeling sorry for yourself. Every salad deserves healthy fats, proteins, and a delicious salad dressing: only then will it sustain you for a whole afternoon, and the nutrients of the salad will be absorbed better. Sprouts are your best buddies—try to add some sprouts to each salad! Carrots contain carotenoid, a phytochemical that can help all kinds of hormonal disorders.

Here's What You Need
2 tablespoons sunflower seeds
2 carrots, finely grated
a piece of fennel, chopped
½ red bell pepper, chopped
about ⅓ cup feta
½ cup broccoli sprouts
a handful of field lettuce (or other green leaves of choice)
½ cup currants

For the dressing

2 teaspoons tahini
1 teaspoon runny honey
½ teaspoon cinnamon
juice of ½ lemon

Here's How You Make It

Roast the sunflower seeds. Roasting reduces the phytic acid and helps with absorption. Make an extra stash for next time. Toss together the carrots, fennel, bell pepper, sunflower seeds, feta, and sprouts. If you eat vegan, replace the feta with cooked beans or quinoa.

Mix together the ingredients for the dressing. Test to see if it still needs anything; make sure you get a good balance between acid and sweet. If you would like it a bit thinner, add water. Line the plate with the green leaves. Scoop the carrot salad in the middle. Drizzle generously with the dressing and toss on some currants.

POINT 2:
DON'T FEAR HEALTHY FATS
(AND EAT THEM!)

WHERE NUTRITION IS concerned, there's a lot of hogwash out there. For decades, we've been told to be frightened of saturated, mostly animal fats because they would be bad for our heart and our blood vessels. And on top of that, we would get fat. Thanks to this the past 40 years have seen an anti-fat campaign, with less and less saturated fats to eat, yet we've been getting fatter and more women have been dying from cardiovascular diseases than from anything else.

IS THERE REALLY A RELATIONSHIP BETWEEN FATTY
FOOD AND CARDIOVASCULAR DISEASE?

It's clear that we've been led down the wrong path. Plenty of research has been done, and more and more doctors confirm it. Anti-fat is now increasingly recognized as a campaign based on little scientific evidence. Despite this new knowledge, the supermarkets are still full of low-fat products. In his book *In Defense of Food*, Michael Pollan points to an article by a group of prominent nutritional scientists at the Harvard School of Public Health. The authors basically pulled the rug from under the fat theory: the vast majority of studies done in this area found no relationship between the consumption of saturated fat and the risk of cardiovascular diseases. Only one strong link has been found between a particular type of fat and heart disease: trans fats. Indeed, these are the fats the food industry has loaded their products with over the past 30 years! The authors concluded that the total fat content in food is of little importance for the risk of heart disease. However, the relationship between the different types of fat is. There are healthy fats, less healthy fats, and unhealthy fats.

During the years of the anti-fat campaign, food manufacturers made our products as fat-free as possible to cater to the desire to eat fats as little as possible. To make up for the loss in flavor, the unwanted fat was replaced by sugars, other sweeteners, and fast carbohydrates, including wheat and trans fats. As it turns out, these are exactly the ingredients that keep you fat and that form the basis of cardiovascular and other chronic diseases!

HEALTHY FATS ARE THE CORNERSTONE OF YOUR HORMONAL HEALTH

The main female hormones, such as estrogen, progesterone, female testosterone, and cortisol, are created from cholesterol, which is a fat. Cholesterol is an essential building block for your female body; that's why your body produces 75 percent of what you require in your liver, leaving about 25 percent that you need to get from your food. This means that it is important to eat healthy fats, along with cholesterol, for healthy cell walls. These cell walls are responsible for good communication in your body and for its being able to quickly recover from stress.

No, You Don't Get Fat from Eating Healthy Fats

It seems contradictory: eat fat but don't get fat. Yet it is not so strange if you use your common sense. Just remember that your body is an organism in which all kinds of complicated processes take place. Butter or other fat is not pasted directly under your skin as extra fat, as if you were plastering a wall. Butter is broken down in your stomach and mixed with acid, after which it is transformed in your intestines with the help of bile, among other things, into all kinds of substances that your body needs. These substances travel from your gut into your bloodstream and from there are transported to the needy cells. Your butter is no longer a fat but has become a building material or energy for your body. There is no direct connection between the butter in your mouth and the fat on your hips. If you think about it like this, then it makes you wonder why we all have believed otherwise for years.

A LOW-FAT DIET DOES NOT REDUCE THE RISK OF CARDIOVASCULAR DISEASES

Two large, long-term health studies are ongoing on women in the United States: the Nurses' Health Study and the Women's Health Initiative.[1] The Nurses' Health Study has collected eating habits and health results of more than 200,000 nurses for decades. The Women's Health Initiative falls under the gold standard in nutrition research: randomized clinical research on a very large group. In this study, the diet and health outcomes of approximately 49,000 women were followed for eight years to see what the effect was of a low-fat diet on the risk of developing breast cancer and cardiovascular diseases, among other conditions. The conclusions of both studies were explosive: a low-fat diet *did not* reduce the risk of cardiovascular diseases.

It is high time to put your fear of healthy fats behind you. Healthy fats are your main energy suppliers, and you need them for a healthy hormone balance. I am convinced that so many women are so tired (and too heavy) because they eat too few healthy fats and are trying to get their energy from sugars and carbohydrates.

CHOLESTEROL IS THE FIRE BRIGADE, NOT THE PYROMANIAC

There is just as much nonsense written about cholesterol as there is about fats. Cholesterol is not your enemy. It is not for nothing that your body creates 75 percent of its cholesterol itself: your body needs it very badly. If you eat too little, your liver makes an extra portion. Your body needs cholesterol as building material for all your cells; without cholesterol, it is not possible to create new cell walls and nerve fibers. Cholesterol is essential for the absorption of vitamins A, D, E, and K. It is also necessary for the production of bile acids. Your brain is full of cholesterol because your brain cells need to communicate with each other. The LDL cholesterol, commonly known as "bad" cholesterol, is the only substance that can bring cholesterol into the mitochondria, the energy factories in your cells. It's not for nothing that healthy fats are our energy suppliers.

Cholesterol Protects You

Elevated cholesterol is not a disease, but it can be a signal that something is out of balance. Usually this is a (chronic) inflammation of the artery walls. Chances are if there's a fire, the Fire Department is there too; this is not to say that the cause of the fire is the Fire Department. It's the same with cholesterol. If there is a raised cholesterol level and inflamed vessel walls, this does not mean that cholesterol is the cause of the problem. Cholesterol is the Fire Department coming to put out the fire.

....

A low-fat diet is an assault on
your health. If you're under stress, your female
body needs healthy fats above all.

....

One of the roles of cholesterol in your body is repairing artery walls. The inflammation in your veins arises not from eating too many healthy fats but from, for example, eating too many bad carbs, sugars, unhealthy fats, wheat products, and processed foods. You require this high cholesterol level to cure the inflammation caused by eating too many of those unhealthy foods.

The use of cholesterol-lowering medicine, therefore, might be similar to sending the Fire Department away. Do you have high cholesterol? Change your diet and see what happens. (Never just stop taking cholesterol-lowering medication; always do this in consultation with your doctor.)

WHAT ARE HEALTHY AND UNHEALTHY FATS?

Healthy fats in the right proportion contain necessary nutrients for your body that you cannot get from another source. They increase the bioavailability of the vitamins and minerals from the rest of your diet. When you add healthy fats, the nutrients are better absorbed in your gut. This makes for a good hormone balance. Also, your brain requires plenty of fats. It consists of 60 percent fats; you keep it healthy by eating healthy fats. Finally, healthy fats stimulate your metabolic rate, so you need them if you want to lose weight.

Very Unhealthy Fats: Trans Fats and Oxidized Fats

It's important to distinguish between healthy fats and unhealthy fats because there are fats that you should avoid as much as possible.

TRANS FATS

Trans fats are artificial fats that are created in a factory by tinkering with liquid plant fats, to make them hard. They are also called hydrogenated fats. Vegetable fats such as corn oil and sunflower oil are naturally fluid. It's hard to use a liquid oil in cookies or puff pastry. Hence, the food industry has changed some molecules in these cheap oils, making them hard. Trans fats are in almost all products that come from a factory, from peanut butter to ice cream, from soups and sauces to chocolate; in bread, crackers, and bouillon cubes and in ready-to-use and fast foods. You consume a lot of trans fats unnoticed, even in the innocent-looking milk powder next to the office coffee maker.

....

Avoid trans fats. They are listed on labels
as hydrogenated fat, hydrogenated oil,
hydrogenated vegetable oil, hydrogenated
vegetable fat, or vegetable oil.

....

OXIDIZED FATS

Oxidation means that the molecular structure of a food changes when it is exposed to light or heat. This change creates free radicals in your body. "Oxidized" means that the product is spoiled. Unfortunately, you often can't see or smell this in fats—they seem to still be fine. Oxidized fats are formed by heating fats that are not appropriate for high heat, such as omega-6 and omega-3 fats. Fried products are full of them. So unfortunately, all chips and deep-fried snacks are on the list of unhealthy fats. If you really want to deep-fry—and my advice is to keep this to a minimum—fry in coconut oil, palm oil, or rice bran oil.

THE REAL BAD GUYS

Trans fats and oxidized fats are known to increase the risk of heart attack. They also burden your liver, which has to rid your body of these unnatural substances. They promote inflammation, hinder the removal of waste substances, and increase your weight, which in turn increases the risk of estrogen dominance. Scientific evidence increasingly shows that they promote insulin resistance and leptin resistance, blood clotting, and diabetes, and can even cause breast cancer. Trans fats and oxidized fats are the real bad guys! Try to avoid them as much as possible. If you don't eat factory-processed foods, you're on the right path.

COCONUT OIL: THE FAT THAT MAKES YOU SLIM

In contrast to other healthy fats, your body cannot create hormones from coconut oil. Nevertheless, coconut oil is a valuable and healthy fat for your kitchen. Coconut fat is solid at room temperature and melts around 35° Celsius (93° Fahrenheit), turning into oil. Coconut fat and coconut oil are the same product. The healthy medium-chain fatty acids in coconut oil are digested very quickly by your body, give energy fast, and are hardly ever stored as fat. In the 1940s, US farmers tried to fatten their cattle with coconut oil. However, the animals became more active and stayed slim. When the farmers switched to soy and corn, the animals got fat again without needing more feed—a fine solution for livestock farmers, but not for you and me.

Coconut Oil Has Many Health Benefits

- Coconut oil contains substances (fatty acids) that fight bacteria, viruses, fungi, parasites, and inflammation. This oil can therefore be deployed to strengthen your intestinal flora or to combat candida or food poisoning.

- Coconut oil can promote better absorption of nutrients from a diseased bowel. This is a benefit for all sorts of intestinal disorders.
- Coconut oil is easily absorbed by the intestines and ensures that all kinds of fat-soluble vitamins, minerals, and proteins are better absorbed. It therefore stimulates your metabolism.
- Coconut oil helps to stabilize your blood sugar, which helps prevent binges during dips in blood sugar levels.
- Coconut contains many antioxidants that protect your body against free radicals. Please note, though: there's a lot of poor-quality coconut oil in circulation. Choose organic extra-virgin coconut oil packed in glass. The coconut smell disappears as it is heated.

The Reasonably Healthy Saturated Fats

Saturated fats are mainly found in animal products such as meat, butter, ghee (clarified butter), and cheese. But palm oil, coconut oil, and cocoa butter also contain saturated fat. Saturated fat is hard at room temperature. The only exception to this is palm oil. Use these fats in moderation; your body doesn't need much. There is one saturated fat that you can use in abundance, and that's coconut oil.

OMEGA-6 FATS: HEALTHY IN MODERATION

Omega-6 fats are found especially in grains, seeds, nuts, and all the oils we produce from them. We often consume too much of these fats because they form the basis of trans fats and are used in the food industry because they are cheap. That is especially true for soybean oil, corn oil, and sunflower oil. Factory-farm animals are fed plenty of soy, corn, and wheat, which means that their products—meat, dairy, and eggs—contain too much omega-6.

CHRONIC INFLAMMATION, YOUR IMMUNE SYSTEM, AND NUTRITION

You may once have had a visible inflammation: say, a splinter in your finger, which over time became red, warm, and swollen. What happens in inflammation is that your immune system tries to drive out the intruder and restore the damaged cells. Inflammation is a protective reaction of your immune system. An acute inflammation is good: your body is healing itself. Chronic inflammation is not healing but destructive. This is also called hidden, silent, or low-grade inflammation, because you don't feel it. Blood tests do not always indicate chronic inflammation.

Women Are More Susceptible to Chronic Inflammation

Any inflammation that lasts longer than 72 hours will slowly poison you. Women are more susceptible to chronic inflammation because we have a more powerful immune system than men against external attackers such as fungi, bacteria, and spoiled food. This powerful immune system can turn against us in the form of autoimmune diseases, a situation in which our immune system can no longer distinguish between enemy cells and our own body cells. Ten times more women than men get autoimmune diseases such as thyroid conditions, MS, rheumatism, Crohn's disease, and Hashimoto's disease.

The Basis of Chronic Disease

Ninety-five percent of all chronic disease is caused by chronic inflammation. Inflammation plays an important role not only in autoimmune disorders but also in cardiovascular diseases, high blood pressure, obesity, insulin resistance, fibromyalgia, depression, osteoporosis, rheumatism, many skin problems, chronic fatigue, and cancer.[2] Chronic inflammation also plays a role in diseases such as

Parkinson's, Alzheimer's, and dementia. More than 80 percent of the cells of your immune system are in your digestive system, in particular in your intestinal flora. Many chronic inflammations start there and are created by the wrong nutrition.

Too much omega-6 can lead to all kinds of chronic inflammation in your body that underlies a wide range of chronic diseases.

Diet Plays an Essential Role in Inflammation

Your diet plays an important role when it comes to the fight against chronic inflammation. Too much omega-6 and saturated fat relative to omega-3 fat is a major cause of chronic inflammation. Further inflammation is caused by all forms of sugars, bad carbohydrates, fructose, chemical additives, artificial sweeteners, gluten, dairy, and arachidonic acid, which is mainly in animal products—all products that are frequently used in processed food from a factory.

All foods that are beneficial for your intestinal flora are also anti-inflammatory. Think of healthy fats (particularly coconut oil, olive oil, and omega-3s), raw foods, vegetables, herbs and spices, and anything with fiber in it, including gluten-free grains and legumes. Eat sufficient vegetable proteins; a healthy immune system needs plenty of protein. I'll get to that in the next chapter.

The Healthy Unsaturated Fats: Omega-3s and Omega-9s

The omega-3 fats are very important for your health; many positive results are attributed to them. Unfortunately, we tend to consume too little omega-3. Omega-3 fats can be found in oily fish such as sardines, salmon, and eel, but also in various vegetable products, such as perilla oil, flaxseed, chia seed, hempseed, and walnuts. Even greens like purslane and watercress contain some omega-3. Omega-9 you'll find mainly in olives, nuts, and avocados.

Omega-3 fatty acids can be divided into three types: ALA (alpha-linolenic acid), EPA (eicosapentaenoic acid), and DHA (docosahexaenoic acid).

YOU SHOULD EAT ALAS

ALA is an essential fatty acid, which means that our bodies cannot create it. We must get it from our diet. ALA is in plenty of plant seeds and oils, particularly in flaxseed, hempseed, canola seed, and walnuts, and therefore also in the oils that are made from them.

EPA AND DHA: EAT THEM
OR MAKE THEM FROM ALAS

The other two fatty acids, EPA and DHA, are especially found in fatty fish, such as salmon, mackerel, sardines, and herring, and also in seaweed and algae. EPA and DHA are powerful anti-inflammatories and can thus protect your joints. They also have positive effects on your immune system and thus on your overall health. In addition, these fatty acids protect your heart, blood vessels, and eyes, and they are important for the proper functioning of your brain in the longer term. There are many health benefits to EPA and DHA.

....

Omega-6s are healthy and you need them, provided you ingest them in the right proportion to omega-3s. The right proportion is 4 times more omega-6 than omega-3. Most people get 20 times more omega-6 because of all the omega-6 in processed food, meat, dairy, and eggs.

....

HOW DO YOU GET OMEGA-3S
IF YOU DON'T WANT FISH?

If you are vegetarian or vegan, then chances are that you ingest too few omega-3 fatty acids. What can you do about it? The good news is that your body can convert ALA into EPA and DHA. That's why vegetarians and vegans choose seeds and nuts and let their bodies do the conversion. The not-so-good news is that this conversion happens rather inefficiently and becomes more difficult as we age. The solution for vegetarians and vegans is to take supplements. Fish oil or krill oil is usually recommended, but you might not want that if you're a vegetarian. Fortunately, nowadays algae oil with high doses of EPA and DHA is available. This is what the fish also eat. Algae-based supplements such as chlorella, spirulina, and marine phytoplankton contain easily absorbable forms of omega-3.

....

Omega-3 is also called our brain food: you need it to keep your brain active. Several studies have shown a relationship between depression and too little omega-3.

....

How Do You Keep Fats Healthy?

You can ruin healthy fats by treating them wrong, such as by heating them or storing them too long outside the fridge. The bad thing is that you often can't see or smell the problem, but they'll no longer be healthy for you—they have become oxidized fats.

HEATING

Heat only coconut oil, palm oil, or rice bran oil. Only these oils are resistant to temperatures of 200° Celsius (390° Fahrenheit) and above. Never fry food in sunflower oil, soybean oil, or corn oil. It gives a boost of free radicals in your body—very good for a few extra wrinkles.

WARMING

Olive oil remains stable to about 160° Celsius (320° Fahrenheit). You can use it to warm food up but not for cooking at high temperatures. The same applies to butter and ghee. Stir-frying with these at low to medium temperatures is fine, but if the oil smokes in your pan, harmful substances arise and you'd better start again. It's better to simmer with these on low heat than fry over high heat. Stir-fry briefly at a high heat only in coconut oil or rice germ oil.

STORING

All vegetable oils from nuts and seeds oxidize when you store them too long or in the daylight. These oils spoil so quickly! Never heat them, and always store them in the refrigerator. Buy them in small dark bottles. Coconut oil and olive oil can be stored outside the fridge.

A Healthy Fats Overview: Omega-3, 6, and 9

Almost all vegetable fats contain a mix of omega-3, omega-6, and omega-9. If you eat a variety of healthy fats, you'll consume all three. First of all, try to eat as much omega-3 as possible, then omega-9, and lastly omega-6. You need all three, but you often consume a lot of omega-6s unnoticed already.

Make Your Own Sauces and Dressings with Healthy Fats

With a nice stock of healthy oils, you can make all kinds of delicious dressings in a snap. Take a good oil plus some lemon juice or good vinegar and some herbs, and you have a delicious dressing. The healthy fats from oil promote better absorption of nutrients. In particular, make your own salad dressing. Most food-industry sauces and dressings are made with the cheapest vegetable oils: sunflower and corn oil, which contain plenty of omega-6 fatty acids. In addition, they contain high doses of sugars, salts, fragrance, colors, and flavors—all substances that create confusion for your hormone balance. They also very often contain the controversial flavor enhancer MSG (E621). You can make much better versions very easily.

SOURCES OF OMEGA-3, 6, AND 9

Sources of Mainly Omega-3s

- perilla oil
- canola oil
- flaxseed and flaxseed oil
- hempseed and hemp oil
- chia seed and chia oil
- walnuts and walnut oil
- organic eggs from free-run chickens
- oily fish such as salmon, mackerel, sardines, and herring—choose the wild varieties: farmed fish eats cereal instead of fish or algae, causing the amount of omega-3 to sharply decrease. Please be aware that approximately 50 percent of the fish currently on offer are farmed.

Sources of Mainly Omega-6s

- sunflower seeds and sunflower oil
- pumpkin seeds and pumpkin seed oil
- sesame seeds and sesame oil
- grapeseed oil
- argan oil
- corn germ oil
- wheat germ oil
- soybean oil
- palm oil
- safflower oil
- peanuts and peanut oil

Sources of Mainly Omega-9s

- olives and olive oil
- hazelnuts, almonds, macadamia nuts, and their oils
- rice bran and rice germ oil
- avocado and avocado oil

AVOID LOW-FAT PRODUCTS—
THEY MAKE YOU FAT AND SICK

The great myth that eating fats makes us fat has led to the appearance of a wide range of low-fat products on supermarket shelves—products with labels stating that they contain less fat or even zero percent fat, as if that's healthy. Not so. In the future, avoid these low-fat products: they usually make you fatter, and sick, too. To give low-fat products a nice mouth feel and make them tastier, the fats are typically replaced with loads of sugars or bad carbohydrates, precisely the ingredients that according to current views are related to weight gain, obesity, diabetes, cardiovascular diseases, and other chronic conditions. They disturb your blood sugar level and increase your chance of insulin and leptin resistance. Be cautious too of packaging that states "low calorie"; usually the sugars have been replaced by chemical sweeteners.

I'm not a fan of dairy, but if there's something healthy about it, it's the fat. Milk is naturally fat, and for good reason. Avoid lean and semi-skimmed milk products; they contain virtually nothing that benefits your body.

A Small Warning

If you add healthy fats to your daily menu, you'll find that you get more satiated. That's a nice feeling. Use it to reduce sugars, carbohydrates, and starches, because those are the substances that actually make you gain weight. Better to eat one slice of bread spread thick with homemade avocado spread than four slices of bread with the same amount of sandwich meat. Eat two or three cups of homemade healthy soup with one slice of bread instead of three slices of bread with a cup of canned soup. Use some raw nuts, seeds, avocado, egg, meat, or fish in every salad, and pour a generous amount of healthy oil with some lemon juice over it. Otherwise, it won't fill you up and you'll be hungry again in a couple of hours.

LIGHT PEANUT BUTTER: 30 PERCENT LESS FAT, 451 PERCENT MORE SUGARS

In 2015, the light peanut butter from the supermarket Plus won third prize from the watchdog Foodwatch. The label mentioned 30 percent less fat, but the fine print showed that a portion of the peanuts had been replaced with corn syrup: there was 451 percent more sugar in it than in normal peanut butter! All supermarkets use the same trick when it comes to "light" products. Don't be fooled: you get fat from sugars, not from healthy fats. Incidentally, peanut butter, to a large extent, contains trans fats, so it's already not so healthy. Peanut butter with a layer of oil floating on it contains no trans fats.

REMEMBER THIS

· Healthy fats are the cornerstone of a healthy hormone balance; your body needs them to create enough hormones.
· Healthy fats are also the basis of your energy management.
· High cholesterol may indicate hidden inflammation in your blood vessels. Cholesterol is not the cause of these infections but the substance that comes to repair the damage.
· In particular, ensure you consume sufficient omega-3 fats. If you don't eat fish, high-quality fish oil, krill oil, or algae supplements are suitable substitutes.
· Heat and warm food only in fats that are suitable for this. Keep other vegetable fats in the fridge to prevent decay.
· Ensure that you have a variety of healthy fats in your kitchen. They will not make you fat.

AVOCADO LEMON TARTS

Having avocados regularly on your menu can boost your health. An avocado is jam-packed with important substances that your body needs. If you are not too fond of them, then I recommend this recipe: this is the way to learn to eat avocado. Never heat avocado, because a big part of the nutrients will be lost.

Because you mix the avocado immediately with the lemon, these tarts stay very green for at least 24 hours. The most delicious nut crusts are those made with organic grass-fed butter. You can also use a high-quality coconut oil, but If you're creating something delicious anyway...

Here's What You Need (for 10 small tarts)

For the crust

½ cup of dried apricots (unsulfured—the dark brown kind)
1 cup of raw nuts
⅔ cup grated coconut
a sprinkle of Celtic Sea salt
2 tablespoons softened grass-fed butter
2- to 3-inch tart tins

For the filling

2 soft dates, pitted
2 avocados
2½ tablespoons maple syrup
3 tablespoons melted coconut oil
the finely ground zest and the juice of 1 lemon
blueberries or shredded coconut (for garnish)

Here's How You Make It

Soak the apricots in hot water for 10 minutes and cut into small pieces. Put them in your food processor with the nuts, grated coconut, and salt and grind into a coarse flour. Add the butter and knead by hand until it forms a sticky dough. Roll out the dough and cut 3- to 4-inch rounds (depending on the size of your tart tin). Line your tart tins with parchment paper and form the dough rounds into little tart shells. Let them set in the refrigerator for about half an hour.

Soak the dates in hot water for 5 minutes. Drain. Put all the filling ingredients except the lemon juice in your food processor and blend to a creamy pudding. Add three-quarters of the lemon juice and blend again. Taste to see if you need the remaining lemon juice—it should be fresh but not too sour. Fill the molds with the filling and put the tarts back in the refrigerator for about an hour. Sprinkle with blueberries or shredded coconut before serving.

8

POINT 3:
EAT AN ABUNDANCE
OF VEGETABLES

I F YOU FOLLOW the points on the Nutrition Compass, chances are you'll belong to the healthiest 5 percent of women. Would you like this? It really isn't difficult. Point 3 shows you the way to eating more plant-based products.

THE RESEARCH THAT COULD HAVE CHANGED THE WORLD

A 5,000-page report from World Cancer Research Fund International published in 2007, to which more than 200 oncologists and scientists contributed and for which thousands of studies were reviewed, showed that if you do not smoke, your diet determines 50 percent of your risk for cancer. If you add your lifestyle (the amount of stress or physical activity you get), you end up with no less than 80 percent.[1] Unfortunately, this research never made the front page of the newspapers, so not many people know about it. The good news from this study is that we have so much influence on our health. This doesn't mean that people who have cancer inflicted it on themselves—there are many more factors we can't control—but nutrition has been shown to be more important than doctors have had us believe.

What Kind of Nutrition Does Your Body Need?

If your diet determines 50 percent of your risk for cancer, then what nutrition does your body need to defend itself in the best possible way against cancer and possibly also all sorts of other chronic diseases? The answer to this question turns out to lie partly in the use of healthy oils and fats and partly in plant products, with vegetables, sprouts, and herbs playing an important role.

IMMIGRATION TO THE WEST INCREASES CANCER RISK

Numerous studies have shown that Asian women are the least affected by breast cancer. When they emigrate to the West, their risk of breast cancer quadruples. This increase is directly linked to changes in their diet.[2]

Give Plants the Lead Role

Thousands of studies have shown that unprocessed plant-based foods, especially vegetables, fruits, seeds, kernels, nuts, seaweed, sprouts, and herbs, play an important role in prevention and cure of cancer and all sorts of other (chronic) diseases. How can that be?

Plants Protect Themselves against Enemies

Plants have their roots in the ground and cannot run away or fight if an enemy such as a fungus or a caterpillar attacks. That is why plants make substances to protect themselves. These substances are called phytochemicals; *phyto* means "plantlike." Research has shown that a large proportion of these substances impede the growth of cancer cells in your body. Vegetables and herbs are the foods with the largest variety of these substances, and give us the most options to reduce the risk of cancer.

Plant Substances Also Protect Your Body

Cabbage- and garlic-type crops contain substances that are able to slow down the growth of cancer cells. Red and purple fruits (such as strawberries, raspberries, and pomegranate seeds) and green tea contain molecules that can prevent micro tumors from forming a network of blood vessels so that their growth is inhibited. Cancer cells are impeded by curcumin, a substance found in the spice turmeric. Ginger and flaxseed can counteract inflammation, giving cancer less opportunity. These are only a few examples out of many. Our daily food contains many cancer-resistant and healing substances.

Plant Fiber Is Important for Healthy Intestines

An additional important advantage of eating a lot of plant foods is that they contain lots of fiber. Fiber matters not only for proper digestion and bowel function, but also for a feeling of satiety. You can eat a lot of this type of food without becoming fat!

Fruit is healthy but does contain fructose. Be cautious with fruit if you regularly feel the need for sweets in any form. Uncontrollable desire to eat sweets or bad carbohydrates means that your blood sugar levels are not yet well balanced. If that's you, choose the more acid forms of fruits, such as grapefruit, sour apples, or sour berries.

Plenty of Vegetables, to Promote Disposal of Xenoestrogens

In Chapter 2 you read about how important it is to make sure that your body disposes of the xenoestrogens you inadvertently ingest. You help your liver with this process by eating plenty of vegetables.

Green vegetables are full of chlorophyll. If your liver has enough chlorophyll, the detoxification process is shortened from seven to two steps. That's why it's smart to make half of your daily vegetables consist of green vegetables.

A DAILY DETOX

Once you add more green vegetables to your daily menu, you make it easier for your body to drain toxins. Detoxification, or detox, is something that you can do every day. It's not as effective to do a detox cleanse twice a year if the rest of the year you're stacking up toxins in your body.

The Four Musketeers: Juices, Soups, Smoothies, and Salads

The biggest change during my burnout happened when I started eating a pound of vegetables a day. You're probably wondering how in heaven's name a person does that, especially when half should be green vegetables. It's not as difficult as you may think. It is, however, a matter of slowly building up to it and letting your body, especially your intestines, get used to it.

I used what I call my Four Musketeers: juices, soups, smoothies, and salads. That's four ways in which you can eat a lot of different vegetables, sprouts, and herbs.

Make juices and smoothies yourself, because everything from the supermarket has lost most of the important nutrients on its way to your kitchen.

Use a slow juicer to make juices and a blender for smoothies. You can have them as breakfast, lunch, or a snack.

Homemade soups with lots of vegetables are very easy to make, and I eat them for lunch, snacks, dinner, or even the next day for breakfast. In Asia, soup for breakfast is very normal. That we need toast for breakfast is also just a habit that somebody once decided was normal. Why not start thinking differently about that now? I eat salads with plenty of vegetables for lunch, snacks, and dinner.

You can, of course, also eat lots of vegetables at dinner. Fill at least half your plate with a variety of colors of vegetables. Each color contains substances that your body needs.

PLANTS CONTAIN NUMEROUS HEALING SUBSTANCES

Thousands of studies have shown that plants contain healing substances. These are exactly the substances used by the pharmaceutical industry. The ancient Greeks already knew that willow bark helped against fever and pain. At the end of the 1800s, scientists discovered this was because of the salicylic acid found in it. They produced a synthetic variety in a laboratory and our aspirin was born. Many substances with plant origins are used by the pharmaceutical industry and turned into drugs.

MAKE ROOM, MAKE ROOM!

If you're going to eat more plant-based products, what would it be wise to eat less of? You have to make room for so many vegetables—your stomach is only so big. What often takes a lot of space on your plate and in your stomach while not adding much to your health?

Eat Meat and Fish in Moderation

Actually, it is a practice out of earlier times to eat so many animal products: for centuries, it was a sign of wealth, showing that you could afford a lot of meat. Eating meat or fish was a status symbol. In developing countries, this is still true. Rich people eat meat and fish; poor people eat little or no meat or fish unless they can catch it themselves or live near water rich in fish, because it is often expensive.

However, the world is changing: in the new world, many people can afford to eat meat and fish daily but choose not to or to do so in moderation, because it's healthier this way—not only for themselves but in other respects too.

Rest assured, I'm not trying to make you a vegetarian. I'm not one: I call myself a vegetarian who occasionally colors outside of the lines. I eat meat and fish, but in moderation. But regardless of your health, which we'll come to in a moment, there are two good reasons to eat less meat and fish.

OUR HEALTH IS LINKED TO THE HEALTH OF OUR EARTH

If we don't keep our earth healthy, our own health will decline. The damage done to our planet by the global livestock industry is enormous. One key cause of the greenhouse effect is the cattle industry. Eighty percent of all agricultural land in the world is for the livestock sector. The large-scale destruction of rain forests is intended to free up more land to grow soy and corn to feed all that livestock. The seas and oceans are being rapidly depleted of fish with nets as big as football fields, 75-mile-long fishing lines, and satellites that can measure exactly where the fish are located. Modern fishing practices mean a lot of technology and little labor. This is an unequal struggle: the fish, and with them our oceans, draw the short straw.

ANTIBIOTICS DO NOT COME ONLY FROM YOUR FAMILY DOCTOR

Eighty percent of all antibiotics produced in the world are given to cattle, chickens, and fish in the meat industry. Antibiotics in your food mean an attack on the health of your gut and your hormone balance.

ANIMAL WELFARE IS FACTORY FARMING'S LOWEST PRIORITY

A second reason to take a second look at eating meat and fish is animal welfare. Unfortunately, we do not live in a world in which animals intended for our consumption are handled properly. They're handled as cheaply as possible, resulting in all kinds of concessions to animal welfare. In addition to the fact that eating lots of meat and fish from factory farms is not healthy for our planet and the animals themselves, we can ask ourselves whether it is good for our own health.

Meat Is Not What It Used to Be

Our grandparents ate meat from animals that ate a lot of natural food and lived outdoors. Cows and other cattle were fed grass and weeds. Pigs are omnivores that are meant to scavenge a wide variety of food from the ground. The same is true for chickens. In the meat industry, however, they are fed cheap soy, corn, or other grains. This has major drawbacks for our health:

- Because these animals are not fed their natural foods, the fat in their meat is full of omega-6 fatty acids instead of the much healthier omega-3s. Omega-6 fatty acids promote inflammation in your body while omega-3s prevent inflammation.
- Corn, soy, and grains intended for feed may be more heavily sprayed with pesticides than those for human consumption. These xenoestrogens enter our bodies through meat.
- Animals in factory farms often receive preventive antibiotics. This is especially the case for pigs and chickens, and it means an extra portion of xenoestrogens on our plates.

Due to all of these practices, the meat of these animals has significantly less nutritional value than it did 30 years ago and also contains contaminants that disrupt your hormone balance. The food industry then adds more:

- Beef looks nice and red because nitrite (E250) is often added. In your body, this substance may be converted into the carcinogen nitrosamine.
- A lot of meat products, such as sausages and pâtés, contain remnants of antibiotics, chemical flavor enhancers, stabilizers, and thickeners. Read the labels. To make meat juicier, phosphates (E450 and E451) are added, which can promote bone loss in humans.
- Frozen meat products are often cheap leftover meats stuck together with meat glue. Meat glue is not really harmful, but do you know exactly what kind of (waste) meat you have on your plate?

Also, the so-called wild game that is offered in the supermarket, such as rabbit or deer, is not really from wild animals that had a good life. This too comes mostly from the meat industry and has the same disadvantages.

....

Nothing has a greater effect on
our earth than what we eat.

....

Our Intestines Are Too Long for Meat

Carnivores in the wild have short intestines because after 24 hours meat begins to rot. By then it should actually already have been excreted. Herbivores in nature have long intestines; plants, nuts, and seeds are difficult to digest and require more time in the intestines to extract all nutrients. People are omnivores: we can eat everything, but in fact, our intestines are a little too long for a lot of meat.

....

Our female intestines are designed
for plenty of vegetable food
with occasional small amounts of meat.

....

To remove meat from your intestines within 24 hours, you need fiber, which is found in plant-based foods. Meat and fish contain no fiber. To eat meat or fish every day and add very little plant-based foods means that there's a lot of rotting food sitting in your intestines.

WOMEN HAVE LONGER INTESTINES THAN MEN

On average, a woman's small intestine is longer than a man's: 7.1 meters (just over 23 feet), compared to 6.9 meters (22 feet). It is believed that this is because it enables women to absorb more nutrients from the intestine during pregnancy. This could also be the reason more women than men suffer from all kinds of stomach and intestinal disorders, including irritable bowel syndrome. It seems as though women's intestines are less suited to meat than those of men.

A CHAT ABOUT POO

A woman who regularly eats meat may have up to 3 kilograms— 6½ pounds—of undigested remnants in her large intestine. That is stuck to the intestinal wall like a paste, causing the passage to become a thin tube. Even if you regularly have diarrhea, you can have this stubborn paste on your intestinal wall. The undigested remnants in this paste contain substances that can be absorbed into your body. This is not harmless: research conducted on this type of intestinal blockage shows that it can contain at least 12 kinds of carcinogens—a good reason to clean your intestines with plenty of fiber from plant-based foods. In addition, you will poop out any overdose of xenoestrogens. Have you eaten a lot of meat for years and now have digestive problems? Then a colonic at a colon hydrotherapist to dispose of this blockage may be a good idea. (Note: Not having a bowel movement every day is also a digestive problem.)

VEINS ARE STIFFER AFTER
A MEAL FULL OF ANIMAL FATS

More women die of cardiovascular disease than of anything else. Research shows that veins become hardened after a meal rich in animal fats. This phenomenon does not occur after eating vegetable fats—vegetable fats are even able to reopen clogged arteries.[3] If you suffer from a heart disease or high blood pressure, it's definitely advisable to eat more vegetable and fewer animal products.

Where Did the Fish on Your Plate Swim?

Fish is easier to digest than meat, so it seems healthier. In addition, it naturally has more of the healthy omega-3 than the omega-6 fatty acids, so this is all good news. But it does matter where your fish comes from. Because wild fish are fewer, there are now large fish farms around the world. About 50 percent of the fish sold, including in boutique fish stores, comes from these farms. Just like a meat producer, a fish producer wants to produce as much fish as possible at the lowest possible cost, which does not benefit our health. Farmed fish, just like cattle, are fed soy and given preventive antibiotics, because the fish are housed too closely together where diseases lurk. Wild fish, of course, do not have these disadvantages, but they increasingly swim in water polluted with chemicals and heavy metals. Larger fish such as tuna and swordfish, which are high in the food chain, can be quite contaminated.

CONSIDER MEAT AND FISH A
TREAT AND CHOOSE ORGANIC

I really wish I could tell a more positive story about eating meat and fish, but for the sake of your health, I cannot and will not pretend that the picture is better than it is. Fortunately, there's a healthy solution: regard meat and fish as a treat, eat it occasionally, buy only the best, purest organic product that you can get, and enjoy it. Choose wild fish, not farmed, when you can. Choose white meat (chicken and turkey) over red meat. In between, eat more plant-based products. Learn to taste again. Organic meat tastes quite different. You'll no longer have to cover up the mediocre flavor with a sauce. Give it a try. If you eat meat or fish, enjoy it. Let quality be more important than quantity. Your health will really benefit.

....

Farmed fish is considered the most
contaminated food on earth.

....

More and more companies and farmers offer honest organic meat, so choosing organic gets easier all the time. If you can't find organic meat or fish near you, try an online frozen organic meat provider.

Meat Substitutes Are the Product of Artful Tinkering

Avoid meat substitutes because virtually all are examples of highly processed artificial food. Vegetable protein must be altered to create a mouthfeel like meat, involving all sorts of products that do not make your body happy and that are full of additives, soy, yeast proteins, and wheat. Organic tempeh is a good choice, though.

HOW DO YOU GET YOUR PROTEIN?

A number of important hormones are made from proteins: insulin, growth hormone, and the thyroid hormones T3 and T4, as well as neurotransmitters such as serotonin, dopamine, and melatonin. Proteins take care of the maintenance and repair of your body. For the construction of all your trillions of new cells you need protein. Eat enough protein: it's important for your hormone balance, but the quality of that protein is also very important. It is often said that we need animal protein and that plant protein is not as good, but that's not so—certainly not for women.

The Eight Essential Amino Acids

Proteins are composed of different amino acids. Your body needs 20 different amino acids to build all kinds of its own proteins, which are necessary for maintaining your various functions. Your body can create most amino acids itself, but there are eight that it must get from your food: these are called the "essential amino acids." Animal proteins contain these eight amino acids; they are found in meat and fish, but also in eggs and dairy products. Proteins from these sources are also called "complete" proteins.

MANY ANIMAL PROTEIN SOURCES ARE LINKED TO DISEASE

A 12-year investigation in which about 90,000 women participated showed that women who ate red meat every day were twice as likely to have breast cancer as women who ate meat less than three times a week.[4] Hundreds of studies have shown that eating a lot of animal protein is linked to conditions common in the West: cardiovascular diseases, cancer, osteoporosis, intestinal problems, obesity, autoimmune disorders, kidney disorders, and diabetes.

When animal proteins are broken down in your body, acids are released. To render these unharmful, your body, among other things, takes calcium from your bones, causing bone loss.

Vegetable proteins come from cereals, legumes, nuts, beans, seeds, seaweed, mushrooms, algae, and vegetables. These proteins are called "incomplete" because in most plant-based products, one or more of the eight essential amino acids is missing.

Full-Fledged Vegetable Proteins

The words "complete" and "incomplete" make it seem as if animal proteins are better. Our ingenious digestive system is, however, perfectly capable of building all necessary amino acids from a combination of plant proteins. Legumes with grains is a familiar combination, but you can also combine pulses with raw nuts, vegetables with sesame seeds, a salad with hemp seeds, a green smoothie with oat milk, or potatoes with eggs. Moreover, you don't need to put these sources of protein on the same plate at the same time. Kidney beans today and brown rice tomorrow is just fine for your body. That makes it a lot easier, doesn't it? If you eat a large variety of plant-based foods, you'll get enough protein. And if you also regularly eat an organic egg, you don't need to worry about the amount of protein at all. Generally, we eat too much protein.

By the way, the idea that plant-based foods never contain all the essential amino acids is outdated. Hemp seeds, quinoa, soy, and spirulina (a type of algae) contain all essential amino acids.

MY PERSONAL TOP 10 VEGETABLE PROTEINS

- hempseed
- quinoa
- tempeh
- vegetables
- legumes
- seeds

- raw nuts
- spirulina
- nutritional yeast flakes
- vegetable protein powder

WOULD YOU LIKE TO CRAVE PHYSICAL ACTIVITY MORE?

Did you know that rats in a laboratory fed a vegetable diet doubled the distance they ran on their treadmills compared with rats on a diet of animal protein? The rats were not rewarded for it. It seemed as if they just enjoyed being more active.[5]

Soy: Healthy for Women or Not?

There is a lot of confusion about the wisdom of soy for women. Is it really a good idea to eat or drink soy, and does it really help with menopause problems? The big disadvantage of soy as we know it is that it is often in the form of milk, yogurt, cream, or desserts, which are all overprocessed. It no longer even resembles soybeans and you often ingest undesirable substances such as fragrance, color, or flavorings. These products are often sweetened and offer no contribution to your health.

Another disadvantage of soy is that it is a goitrogen substance, which may have a harmful effect on the thyroid gland. Soy can exacerbate iodine deficiency, and you need iodine to keep your thyroid functioning well. A quarter of women over 45 suffer from a slow thyroid—more reason to be careful with soy.

Soy products sometimes contain, as a residual of the production process, aluminum, which is toxic to your nervous system and kidneys. One constituent of soy is phytic acid. The problem with phytic acid is that it obstructs the absorption of essential minerals such as calcium, magnesium, iron, copper, and zinc from your gut. Women need enough iron throughout the years they menstruate. Eating soy products limits the efficacy of B12 (iron) and vitamin D. So soy is really not that healthy.

The positive story of soy for women revolves around the fact that it contains phytoestrogens. Phytoestrogens (*phyto* means "plant"), like xenoestrogens, mimic the estrogen in your body. What makes phytoestrogens interesting is that they are adaptogenic. This means that they do regulatory work. If your estrogen level is too low, they increase it, which is fine. If your estrogen level is too high, they block the estrogen receptors, so that your estrogen or the even more powerful xenoestrogens lose access. This helps reduce your estrogen level. Phytoestrogens create a balance in your endocrine system.

However, what few women know is that phytoestrogens are released only when soy is fermented. Asians have found a way to ferment soybeans which makes them healthy. Think of products such as miso, tamari, tempeh, natto, and fermented soy sauce (tofu is unfermented soy). The phytic acid in fermented soy is broken down. These are good products. Choose organic options when you can, and as pure as possible.

Instead of fermented soy, you can also use freshly ground flaxseed to balance your estrogen. This contains the same phytoestrogens (lignans) as soy. Overall, the evidence seems to indicate that it's best to avoid or consume very little soy, with the exception of fermented soy products.

REMEMBER THIS

- Plants contain all kinds of healthy and healing substances. Eat the widest possible variety of plant-based products.
- Our intestines are slightly too long for a lot of meat. Plants contain plenty of fibers that are important for healthy intestines.

- Nonorganic meat and fish contain substances that can upset your hormone balance. Eat less meat and fish, and when you do eat them, choose organic and the highest possible quality.
- There are plenty of opportunities to get proteins from plant-based products.

VEGETABLE SALAD WITH GRATED EGG

Your liver desperately needs green vegetables, preferably combined with proteins. That is why I regularly put a hearty green salad on the table. This is my favorite green vegetable salad, with a delicious mustard-dill dressing. You can replace the tamari almonds with pieces of (organic) chicken or crumbled feta.

Here's What You Need (for 2 servings)
4 large organic eggs
Celtic Sea salt
fresh pepper
5 large spears green asparagus
1 cup broccolini (from the broccoli family)
1 cup sugar snap peas
⅓ cup peas (can be from frozen)
2 tablespoons tamari almonds (see the recipe for tamari Brazil nuts, page 95)

For the dressing

1 tablespoon grapefruit juice
2 tablespoons extra-virgin olive oil (flaxseed oil is fine too)
1 teaspoon mustard
1 teaspoon honey
1 tablespoon fresh or dried dill

Here's How You Make It
Place the eggs in a small pot on the stove. Top them with boiling water and let them boil 6 minutes. Drain and rinse with cold water. Peel and grate the eggs finely on a sharp grater. Sprinkle generously with salt and pepper.

Make the dressing by mixing all the ingredients together. Taste to see what else it needs.

Remove the hard ends of the green asparagus. Cut 2 inches under the tops and cut the bottom portion into two pieces. Cut it in half lengthwise. Do the same with the broccolini: leave the tops whole but cut the stalks in half. Small pieces cook quickly. Trim the sugar snaps.

Place the sugar snaps in a steamer over boiling water and steam for 1 minute. (If you do not have a steamer, place the vegetables in a large pot with a little boiling water. Let them simmer.) Add the asparagus and broccolini and let this cook about 5 minutes. When the vegetables are almost tender, add the peas. Cook 1 more minute. Spoon the vegetables directly onto the plates. Add the eggs and the dressing and, lastly, sprinkle with the chopped tamari almonds.

9

POINT 4:
BE SMARTER THAN SWEETS

NTIL PUBERTY, SWEETS were not a problem for me. I loved chocolate and other sweet things, but I didn't think all the time about eating candy; there were plenty of other fun things to do. In my adolescence, I gained the predictable female pounds and it wasn't long before I thought that it was more than a good thing. One day, when someone casually mentioned that I had grown a tummy, I'd had enough—and I immediately started on a diet! This was the beginning of a very long period of starving interspersed with binging on sweets.

SUGAR ADDICTION IS NOT LACK OF WILLPOWER

If only someone had told me then about the addictiveness of sugar and how women especially crave it! The only thing I could think of was that I just had no willpower and that everyone dealt with treats normally except me: I regularly emptied a tin of chocolate cookies instead of eating a plate of hot food.

Only now do I understand that my sugar addiction had nothing to do with willpower or lack of perseverance. I just didn't know how strongly my body was programmed to find sugar tasty (especially in combination with fats and some salt) and how many products from the food industry have deliberately been created to have such a strong addictive effect. I also didn't know that it was my female endocrine system, with fluctuating estrogen levels, that caused me to regularly grab sweets like a junkie, especially in the days just before getting my period.

If only I'd known all of that sooner, I wouldn't have been so down on myself and kept myself small. That's why I want to tell you this. If you know how it works, it's not so hard to be smarter than sugar.

....

A sugar addiction in particular can cause women to eat too little healthy food.

....

Your Body Is Programmed to Find Sweets Tasty

Nature gives us sugars only in summer and early autumn. Summer sees a variety of red fruits, such as berries, strawberries, and cherries, while apples and pears ripen in the fall along with beets, carrots, potatoes and other tubers, which behave like sugar in our body. Nature had a reason for this. Sugars, carbohydrates, and starches are meant to be tasty and give us a layer of fat. After you eat them, your body makes insulin, and as long as insulin is circulating in your blood, your body doesn't burn fat. It used to be vitally important that we entered the winter with a layer of fat, because in the winter, there was considerably less food available. This layer of fat was especially essential for women who became pregnant or who were breastfeeding. Hence, women store fat more easily than men (and have more trouble getting rid of it again): for the survival of humanity, women had a layer of fat. Sugar is an essential part of our bodies' survival mechanism.

WOMEN BECOME ESPECIALLY ADDICTED

It's not only the delicious taste in your mouth that is addictive. There's more to the story. When you eat sweets, the hormone dopamine is generated in your brain and gives you a flood of good feeling. This calls for more. And this is why a lot of food is so addictive. You can read more about this in Chapter 6. The addictiveness of processed foods is hugely underestimated. Women in particular are at a disadvantage.

Overeating Triggers Your Brain to Eat More and More Food

Research shows that women are twice as likely to become addicted to food as men.[1] Women diet more, with the result that we often do not eat enough, and if we don't persevere (and in 98 percent of cases, we fail), we alternate that with overeating. We do that mostly with sweets, bad carbs, or something that contains the addictive combination of sugar, fat, and salt. No one overindulges on broccoli or celery.

Compulsive eating works like cigarette addiction: no one becomes addicted after smoking one cigarette. The addiction starts if you're a regular, smoking one or more cigarettes every day. The need for nicotine then grows larger and larger. No addict started with two packs per day, but the body craves more to get that satisfied feeling. The same is true for drugs and addictive food. Your sense of satiety becomes dulled if you overeat every time, especially when eating sugars. You'll need more sugars next time to get the same feeling.

BREAST MILK IS SWEET

Breast milk is sweet. It's supposed to be, so that the baby drinks it easily and gains weight. We're programmed to like anything sweet.

....

Alternating between getting too little
food and overeating triggers your brain, making
it more and more addicted to overeating, so
that you'll need more and more food.

....

Low Estrogen Levels Can Make You Crave Sweets

As a woman, you don't wrestle only with the addictiveness of processed food. There's also your hormones causing you to eat too much. Do you get a strong need for certain foods, often sweets, before your period? Hormone fluctuations just before your period can make you take leave of your common sense.

NOT EATING ENOUGH WILL SOONER OR LATER RESULT IN A BINGE

Always trying to lose a few (or many) pounds and therefore not eating enough will sooner or later result in a binge, because your body can no longer trust that it will regularly receive enough nutrition. That distrust leads not only to cravings, but also to the storing of fat from the foods that you do eat and the slowing down of your metabolism, by which you gain weight.

HUNGRY BEFORE YOUR PERIOD?

Professor Kelly Klump examined the relationship between menstrual cycle and hunger.[2] During ovulation, few women felt the need to binge. The period after ovulation until menstruation turned out to be when many women tended to lose control of their eating. As menstruation approached, this was felt ever more strongly. The cravings disappeared on the day of menstruation.

....
It's incredible how our hormones can persuade us to eat sweets!
....

Estrogen Influences Your Brain

In the days before your period, the hormone estrogen drops to make way for progesterone. Estrogen has a direct impact on the opiate-producing centers in your brain. Dopamine and serotonin are the opiates stimulated by estrogen, and they make you feel good and peaceful. The low estrogen level before your period can lead to lower levels of serotonin and dopamine. This doesn't feel good—it makes you uneasy, you get unexplained mood swings, and you can feel depressed or even anxious. These are the moments when your body starts to crave food and especially sweets: sweets also stimulate the production of dopamine and serotonin. However, sweet foods make the problem worse.

PMS: An Insatiable Monster in Search of Food?

PMS stands for "premenstrual syndrome." PMS complaints are those that occur prior to menstruation, and they may get worse as you age. They can also begin in perimenopause. Physically, these are the most common symptoms: sore breasts, bloating, water retention, sleep problems, migraines, headaches, and muscle and joint pain. Some of the emotional issues are binge eating and strong cravings for sweet foods, emotionality, irritability, fatigue, changing moods, depression, and even aggression.

The degree of your PMS problems, including hunger, depends on the extent to which your hormones are in balance with each other. The balance between estrogen and progesterone plays an important role. From around the age of 35, that balance can fluctuate strongly before your period. It can, as a client of mine said, turn you into "an insatiable monster that is constantly looking for chocolate."

Research has shown that women with PMS have low serotonin levels. Serotonin, the happiness hormone, is the substance that makes you feel good. A low serotonin level can give rise to emotions like irritability, or to anxiety or depression. This is caused by estrogen levels being too low. Eating sweets or bad carbohydrates will temporarily boost serotonin levels. This is why your body longs for junk. The problem, however, is that eating sweets is a solution that only makes the situation worse in the long term.

The reason: inflammation from fluctuating blood glucose levels. The cause of PMS seems to lie in cellular inflammation that results from a fast-rising blood sugar level. The only solution for PMS symptoms is to keep your blood glucose levels as stable as possible. If you find this difficult in the days before your period, then at least try it in the weeks after. The better you manage to keep your blood glucose level stable during this time, the fewer or less extreme PMS symptoms you will get. Just remember that there are multiple things other than sweets that cause your blood sugar levels to peak; see the table in Chapter 2 (page 65).

A SMART WAY TO KEEP YOUR
BLOOD GLUCOSE LEVEL STABLE

The glycemic load (GL) of any food is the effect that the food has on your blood glucose levels, as measured by a normal portion. A high GL means a higher peak. Dried fruit has a very high GL, vegetables a low one. Many books give tables with the GL of foods and advise you to avoid the foods with a high GL. But it's also important to look at nutritional value. There are foods with a high GL that contain plenty of healthy nutrients, such as fruit; we should keep eating these. A smart way to eat these healthy high-GL foods without causing a peak in your blood glucose level is by combining them with healthy fats, proteins, fibers, and/or certain herbs. This works as follows...

Here's How You Keep Your Blood Sugar Stable

If you eat something that consists mainly of sugars or bad carbohydrates, your blood glucose levels peak. A smoothie made only from fruit or a slice of bread with jam can be transported from your stomach to your gut relatively quickly, which will lead to a quick peak. If there are fats in the food mash in your stomach, then your liver first has to create bile before the mash can pass into your intestines. The bile will take care of the breakdown of fats. Bile is made little by little by your liver and transported to your stomach. The food mash, therefore, also moves little by little from your stomach to your intestines. A food mash with fats remains in your stomach much longer than a mash without fats, and will cause less of a blood sugar peak. An additional advantage is that you have a longer sense of satiety because it takes longer before your stomach is empty. Much the same is true for proteins, fibers, and certain spices—they also slow down this process.

Slap half an avocado on your sandwich or add a thick piece of wild salmon or a boiled egg with a layer of coconut oil underneath it. This is better for your blood sugar level, and thus for your weight, than a slice of bread topped with tomato and cucumber. Again: don't be afraid of healthy fats! They are your best friends. The same is true for pasta, whole grain rice, and sweet potatoes: eat a little pasta but with lots of fresh tomato sauce full of vegetables and some olives. Eat a little whole grain rice and a lot of that homemade curry with all sorts of vegetables and coconut cream, and eat a baked sweet potato with a big helping of a green salad loaded with nuts and dressing. Don't leave the fats out of the recipes in this book; you need them.

Thousands of studies have shown the harmful effects of prolonged (high) sugar consumption. The problem for women in particular is that sugars cause a serious imbalance in our sensitive endocrine system. Aside from the negative influence on your blood sugar level, with the possible consequence of obesity, insulin resistance, leptin resistance, and type 2 diabetes, there are even more reasons for you as a woman to significantly reduce sweet things in your life:

....

Would you like more life in your life?
A higher quality of life? Get rid of sugar.

....

- Overproduction of insulin disturbs other hormones in your body. Too much insulin can cause your female testosterone to rise, and you may break out in pimples and male hair growth patterns. This is an increasingly common phenomenon called polycystic ovary syndrome (PCOS).
- Sugar upsets the mineral balance in your body and depletes your bones of calcium and magnesium, with resulting bone loss.
- All forms of sugars rob your body of vitamins and minerals, especially B vitamins and magnesium. Your body needs these vitamins and minerals to store sugars as energy for later use. The B vitamins give you that energy, and magnesium is a mineral needed for many of your body's processes. Many women who complain of fatigue are low on magnesium and B vitamins.
- Cancer feeds on sugars. A high sugar intake raises the risk of breast cancer, colon cancer, and cardiovascular diseases.
- Excessive sugar has an impact on your brain. It overstimulates endorphins, making you restless, irritable, and anxious. It can lead to concentration problems, a foggy feeling in your head, depression, and lethargy.
- Diseases such as Parkinson's and Alzheimer's, which are becoming more common in younger women, are partly attributed to our high sugar consumption.
- Excess sugar is converted into fatty acids, thus increasing the chance of arteriosclerosis. This can lead to strokes or

heart attacks. The largest cause of death among women is cardiovascular disease.

· Too much sugar disrupts your immune system, creating hidden inflammations, large and small, in your body. Hidden inflammation is the cause of all kinds of chronic diseases.

· Your intestinal flora is disturbed by an overabundance of sugars. This encourages the growth of candida in your intestinal flora. If this yeast turns into a fungal infection, it can do all kinds of damage to your body.

· Ninety percent of your happiness hormone, serotonin, is created in your gut. Disruption of your intestinal flora from too much sugar means you keep grabbing for sweets out of frustration or feelings of displeasure.

· Too much sugar, and thus higher insulin production, causes premature aging.

"LIGHT" PRODUCTS MAKE YOU FAT AND SICK

You've already read in Chapter 7 that skim milk products are not healthy because the fats have almost always been replaced by sugars. The same goes for "light" products, in which the sugars have been replaced by artificial sweeteners. Do you use sweeteners in your coffee, drink diet cola, and grab "light" products because you want to lose weight? Then I have bad news for you: these products are even worse for you and your healthy weight than the occasional bit of sugar. Scientists have developed a whole range of synthetic sweeteners that can replace sugars. These include sorbitol, xylitol, isomalt, processed stevia products, sucralose, saccharin, aspartame, and cyclamate. They contain no calories and are therefore used to sweeten "light" products.

"Light" Products Are Also Addictive

We tend to eat or drink "light" foods in greater quantities because they contain no calories—so you take another diet cola. But it's not so simple. The more you use, the more you need these products for your sugar kicks and temporary good feeling. "Light" products are also addictive. One study found that the sweetener saccharin is no less than eight times as addictive as cocaine.[3] But that's not all. A 14-year study of 66,000 women showed that women who used these products became heavier and sicker than women who used products made without artificial sweeteners but with regular sugar. Diabetes risk was greater in women who consumed "light" drinks. These women also suffered more sugar cravings, making them eat more sweets or pasta or bread for dinner, and so were heavier.[4] Many studies have revealed that users of "light" products increase their risk of being overweight by as much as 200 percent! This is because these products fool your metabolism. Several things go wrong in your body when you use these chemicals.

SWEETENERS CAN INCREASE WEIGHT BY 25 PERCENT

Studies of rats showed that they ate more calories if they were given small amounts of artificial sweeteners than did the control group, who were given regular sugars. In one study, the rats fed artificial sweeteners were shown to be as much as 25 percent heavier after just one month.[5]

....

Because "light" products disrupt your body
with chemicals, your body can no longer make
a good assessment of how much food it
needs, and the chance of overeating is very large.

....

"Light" Products Fool Your Body

Light products disrupt your sense of hunger and satiety. Your body thinks it's getting energy (because it's consuming something sweet), but it doesn't get that energy in the form of glucose. It's fooled and goes on a search for all that energy. This is the cause of the craving for sugars and carbohydrates that often results after eating or drinking "light" products. On top of that, almost all artificial sweeteners are synthetic products that your body doesn't recognize and that it then has to dispose of. This means an overload for your liver.

What Are Healthier Sweeteners?

To sweeten, I choose maple syrup, raw agave, amazake, coconut blossom sugar, or raw honey, depending on the recipe. Also dates, apricots, and other sweet dried fruit can provide a sweet taste to your dish. Your body recognizes these sweeteners. They contain some natural minerals and nutrients, but use them in moderation and, even then, as much as possible in combination with fats, proteins, or herbs that prevent your blood glucose level from having too many peaks. See Appendix A for more healthy alternatives. Keep in mind that the only way to get rid of your urge for sweets is to use less and less of them.

WHAT SHALL WE DO WITH ALCOHOL?

In this chapter on sugars, I cannot avoid alcohol: alcohol is also a form of sugar. Don't worry—I'm not a prohibitionist. I like a glass of wine. I know that no alcohol at all would be better for me, but I really enjoy wine in good company. And as I enjoy it, my body makes endorphins and hormones that are healthy for me, or so I like to think. But I know that I'm giving my liver extra work with that glass of wine. That's why I pay attention to what it does to me, and I find myself increasingly leaving it alone. I put the bar for my vitality and good health high, so I'm feeling less and less inclined to take that glass of wine.

Women Are More Susceptible to Alcohol Addiction

I do understand that women can lose themselves in alcohol. Especially when you feel emotionally cold, alcohol can seem like a delicious, warm blanket. You may feel it seems to help you relax after the day's stress, to make you forget your worries or challenges, and to be a good friend if you're at home alone on the couch on a Friday evening. I know all about that!

Everything I've written about what sugar does, however, also applies to alcohol. As with sugars, women are also more susceptible to alcohol addiction than men. Drinking alcohol seems to give a temporary moment of relaxation, but from the first sip, you give yourself a lot of extra work: alcohol means stress for your body. Alcohol immediately increases your cortisol level, because all sorts of things must happen to get it out of your body again.

Alcohol Aggravates Estrogen Dominance

Alcohol also causes an increase in your estrogen level, and thereby increases estrogen dominance with all its consequences. In addition, alcohol works like a diuretic, which will flush out all kinds of valuable vitamins and minerals from your body. Even if you've banished toxins from your life as much as possible, it's still not a good idea to get wasted on the weekend or drink a glass of wine every night.

Don't Drink on an Empty Stomach

Don't have that glass of alcohol on an empty stomach—you'll feel it that much more. Your blood glucose level certainly won't be happy with it, so if you want to lose weight, alcohol is the first thing you might look at critically. If you do drink alcohol at a dinner party, eat plenty of vegetables or other fibers. Drink two glasses of water for every glass of alcohol to compensate for the fluid that you lost. Dry mouth and a headache after an evening of heavy drinking are a result of alcohol dehydrating your body. Coffee is also a diuretic, so having coffee the next morning to cure your hangover is a really bad plan.

What about Red Wine?

If you enjoy wine like I do, you've probably been pleased to read that red wine is not so bad. The grape peel used when making red wine contains resveratrol, which is a powerful antioxidant. Grapes still on the vine use resveratrol to keep fungi at a distance. This story, however, applies to only organic red wine, because antifungal chemicals are used on nonorganic grapes, which will make less resveratrol as a result. Grapes for wine are plentifully sprayed, so organic wine is always a healthier choice than nonorganic. This also applies to white wine. Unfortunately, there's no resveratrol in white wine because the peel is not used.

Here too it is wise to choose quality. Choose a good organic (red) wine and enjoy it! Do you drink other alcoholic beverages? Anything is okay once, but think of it as a treat and drink in moderation. Check your energy levels the morning after and ask yourself whether it was worth it.

And a Beer?

Be careful with beer if you're struggling with your weight. Men who drink a lot of beer don't get beer bellies for nothing. Beer is made from grain and contains maltose, a type of sugar that causes your blood glucose level to rise like a rocket. Beer also contains hops; hops contain powerful phytoestrogens that can cause extra storage of fat around your waist and breasts.

PLEASE DON'T TOUCH MY COFFEE

Are you a true coffee drinker? Many women are exhausted and crave coffee due to an overload of stress and a lack of sleep. I had a client who drank 20 cups of black coffee a day just to keep going. No wonder she couldn't sleep at night and struggled with her weight! Yes, even black coffee without sugar can make you fat, because it affects your blood glucose level.

What happens in your body when you drink a cup of coffee? The caffeine will give you a boost. As soon as the first sip of coffee ends up in your stomach, there's a call to your adrenal glands that they have to create extra cortisol. Drinking coffee while you're already under a lot of stress is therefore a duplication. And if you also eat a lot of sugars or bad carbs, the effect is tripled. All three spike your blood sugar level, and in all three cases, insulin is created. Do you remember the table from Chapter 2? That table could also be labeled "How Can I Make My Waist a Fat Magnet?" An overdose of coffee, sugars, and stress can also lead to sleep problems, and if there's one thing that's good for your health, your energy levels, and maintaining a healthy weight, it's a good night's sleep.

Caffeine Isn't Just in Coffee

Caffeine is not found only in coffee. It's also in chocolate, black tea, white tea, green tea, and some soft drinks, including colas and energy drinks. Soft drinks and energy drinks in particular consist of an overdose on sugars (one can might contain the equivalent of over 20 sugar cubes!) in combination with caffeine or another stimulant. That will give you an energy boost in the short term, but in the longer term, it ensures a blood sugar crash: mood swings, brain fog, a headache, and a craving for sweets again.

Two Cups a Day Is Okay

You don't have to quit completely, because a cup of coffee or two a day is not that bad. Research even shows that coffee contains plenty of healthy substances that can reduce the chance of Alzheimer's, Parkinson's, or a stroke. It's not the caffeine that provides this but other substances in the coffee beans. Are you sleeping poorly? Then drink coffee in the morning, not past noon. A good substitute for coffee is any type of herbal tea. It comes in dozens of flavors. Figure out what your favorites are and vary them regularly. Do you feel that you need a caffeine boost? Choose green or white tea, which contains theine, similar to caffeine.

HAVE YOU HEARD OF COCONUT COFFEE?

Stir a teaspoon of coconut oil into your coffee. Coconut oil is directly converted into energy by your body, not stored as fat. Your brain gets an immediate boost!

Need an afternoon pick-me-up?
Try replacing that cup of coffee with some deep breaths and a glass of water.

NEED A BOOST?

Do you need a quick boost? Then get your body moving for a few minutes! Walk quickly up and down a few flights of stairs, jump rope for a minute, open a window and take 20 deep breaths, making sure you fill your belly. Do 10 push-ups or jumping jacks, or create something yourself to make you feel the blood flowing through your veins again. End with two large glasses of clean, vital water and you can get at it again. Even without coffee.

Decaf Is Not the Solution

Do you panic at the idea that you should drink less coffee? It's not considered an addictive substance for nothing. Wean yourself slowly. Coffee without caffeine is not the solution, though. The disadvantage of many kinds of decaffeinated coffee is that a chemical process is used to remove the caffeine. These chemicals get in your body via the coffee. A different process is used for organic decaffeinated coffee, so that is a good choice.

BE SMARTER THAN SUGAR

You don't always have to say no to everything; your body needs a small serving of healthy sugars every day. What matters is that you get back in control and are not a slave of the food industry or of your hormones. Don't fight sugars, but make sure you're smarter than them. How do you do that?

Nourish Yourself with Plenty of Healthy Food

First feed yourself well, then leave out less healthy things: that's the basis of the Nutrition Compass. That is why omitting sugars isn't till Step 4. The need for sugars is often a need for energy, which your body can get only from healthy food. Feeding yourself well with all kinds of healthy, natural products is therefore the best remedy for a sugar addiction. It will decrease the need for sugars.

Let Your Taste Buds Help You

The good news is that your taste buds are going to help you with this. Every two weeks, the cells of your taste buds are renewed. If you manage to avoid eating sweets for two weeks, you'll notice that you're going to find many things too sweet, especially the highly processed factory foods. You'll notice that store-bought products like mayonnaise, spaghetti sauce, and peanut butter are sweetened, and believe it or not, you'll find them less and less tasty. Every woman who has recovered from an overdose of sweetness will agree.

Don't Skip Breakfast

An uncontrollable desire for sweets often arises if your blood glucose level dips, so don't skip breakfast, certainly not as long as your blood glucose level is fluctuating. With breakfast you establish the basis for your blood glucose level for the rest of the day. Make sure you get a good balance of protein, healthy fats, and some slow carbohydrates.

Choose Healthy Snacks

If you're in need of sweets, drink two large glasses of water. Your brain knows no difference between hunger and thirst. Chances are your body is thirsty, not hungry. If you still have a craving, eat something that's not too sweet and preferably that also contains healthy fats and proteins. Some raw nuts or a soft-boiled egg is fine. Combine this with some fruit if you feel that your body really needs sugar. A piece of fruit together with some raw nuts is a great snack. Make sure you always have a healthy snack on hand in case you need something. A green, not too sweet, smoothie is ideal, because you can always take it with you. You don't have to completely wean off sweets quickly. You control the pace—just make sure you're heading in the right direction.

TEN HEALTHY WAYS TO GIVE YOUR FEEL-GOOD HORMONES A BOOST

Do you often grab sweets because you want to feel better? There are plenty of healthier ways for you to give your feel-good hormones a boost. If you use them regularly, you'll soon be able to notice the difference.

1. GIVE YOURSELF A TRYPTOPHAN BOOST.

The raw material of the happiness hormone serotonin is an amino acid called tryptophan. The more tryptophan your body gets, the more serotonin it can create. Tryptophan is found in, among other things, chia seeds, sesame seeds, sunflower seeds, oats, oat bran, buckwheat, raw organic protein, chestnuts, basil, spirulina, tempeh, Parmesan cheese, and poultry. Tryptophan is also the raw material of the sleep hormone melatonin, so if you sleep badly, these foods can also help you.

2. EAT HEALTHY CARBOHYDRATES.

Replace eating sweets and bad carbohydrates with healthier forms of sweets and carbohydrates, which will give you the same serotonin and dopamine boost. Choose unprocessed products that won't make your blood glucose level peak too quickly. Consider bananas, blueberries, gluten-free pasta, an almond milk smoothie, buckwheat pancakes, or home-baked muffins or cake.

3. ENJOY HEALTHY CHOCOLATE.

Chocolate makes many women feel good. This isn't just because it tastes so good, but also because there are many healthy nutrients in it, including tryptophan, theobromine, and magnesium. Choose healthy chocolate. Eat chocolate with at least 70 percent cocoa or, even better, make healthy raw cacao treats and be sure to always have a few in your freezer.

4. GET PLENTY OF NATURAL LIGHT.

There is a clear relationship between lack of daylight and depressive feelings. Thanks to daylight, your skin makes vitamin D. Vitamin D is actually a hormone that controls many functions in your body. You can't get enough from your diet every day, so a dose of daylight can certainly help.

5. GET MOVING.

Do you need a quick boost of feel-good hormones? Put your body in motion. At least 20 to 30 minutes every day of good physical activity (brisk walking or cycling, trampoline jumping, strength training) gives your body an extra portion of endorphins. If you do that outdoors, you also get a dose of natural light. Find a form of exercise that you like, so that it gives you some joy every day.

6. ALLOW YOURSELF ADEQUATE REST AND SLEEP.

There are few things that rob you of good feelings more than fatigue. If you feel exhausted during the day, feel free to plan a power nap.

Twenty minutes' sleep can boost your hormones. Or plan a long evening in for yourself. Let everyone know you're not available. Take a bath with lavender and magnesium (Epsom salts), let yourself relax, and dive in your bed with a good book.

7. SURROUND YOURSELF WITH KINDNESS.

Research shows that being kind to someone gives your serotonin levels a boost. The interesting thing is that the same study found that not only the giver but also the recipient got this serotonin boost.[6] If you're the one who is always kind and caring to others, make sure the roles are sometimes reversed. Even watching people be friendly to each other gives your feel-good hormones a boost. In short: surround yourself with kindness and stay away from people who quarrel.

8. JUMP AROUND, AND FAKE IT TILL YOU MAKE IT.

We can influence our brain and emotions with our bodies. Just try to feel depressed while you're skipping or smiling! If our body radiates joy or does something related to excitement, our brain apparently thinks that we're really enjoying ourselves. Skip regularly or watch videos or movies that make you laugh. It really helps!

9. CUDDLE AND PLAY ALWAYS HELP.

Hugging is a great way to make yourself feel better. Just ask your loved ones for a hug if you feel it will do you good. Or maybe a pet is what you need? There is much research showing that having a pet can be very healthy for us. Playing with pets and cuddling them in particular makes us feel good.

10. BE GRATEFUL.

If you're feeling down, it's not always easy to feel grateful for what you do have. Still, it's a very good way to make yourself feel a little better. In your mind, go back to a time when you felt truly grateful. Experience this moment again and let this emotion well up in you. Your body will respond to this by recreating the hormones that belonged to that moment. No matter how many setbacks you have, there are always little things in your life for which you can be grateful.

REMEMBER THIS

- We can become powerfully addicted to sugars, especially in combination with fats and some salt, like we can to opium or cocaine.
- Women become more easily addicted to overeating than men do.
- A fluctuating estrogen level can cause extreme hunger or the need for sweets. Low estrogen levels will send you to seek nutrients.
- The largest amounts of sugar are hidden in factory-processed foods. Many drinks, including fruit juices, are liquid sweets.
- "Light" products are not a solution: their chemicals disrupt your body, including your hormone balance.
- Drink alcohol in moderation—no more than two drinks per day, and preferably no more than two days a week. Pay close attention to what it does to you.
- Drink coffee in moderation, especially if you're under a lot of stress or are addicted to sweets. Don't drink more than two cups a day, preferably in the morning.
- Eating candy makes you feel good, but there are healthier ways to achieve this good feeling.

RAW OATMEAL WITH ORANGE JUICE

Rolled oats are very nutritious and contain plenty of fiber. That helps keep your blood sugar level balanced and ensures healthy intestinal flora. Oats also contain a lot of tryptophan, the raw material of serotonin. Serotonin will help you feel good and therefore help you control your cravings for sweets.

Not everyone knows that you don't have to cook rolled oats. You can also eat them raw. It's a good idea to let them soak overnight to help break down the phytic acid, which can hinder the absorption of vitamins and minerals in your intestines. I like to soak them in orange juice and make breakfast the next day with anything that I have on hand, such as fresh fruit sprinkled with some Energetic Woman's Granola—very simple, and very healthy. You can take this breakfast with you in a tightly sealed canning jar.

Here's What You Need
2 tablespoons rolled oats
the juice of 1 orange
a mix of fresh and dried fruits, nuts, seeds, and kernels

Here's How You Make It
Put the rolled oats in a glass canning jar. Squeeze the orange, then mix the juice and the flesh from your citrus press with the oats. Let this sit overnight, covered or uncovered; if the room is warm, make that be in the fridge. Next morning, stir it well and sprinkle with some combination of fresh fruit, dried fruit, seeds, nuts, or healthy granola.

10

POINT 5:
COW'S MILK IS FOR CALVES

NOW COME TO a topic that can be quite sensitive, because just as there are women calling out "Don't touch my coffee!" so too are there women who are very unhappy if you mess with their daily bowl of fruit yogurt or chunk of cheese. It can't be that bad, can it? It comes from a cow and is a natural product?

However, I'm going to explain why eating and drinking a lot of dairy is not such a good idea for the health of your gut and your hormones. It might even be a very good idea to avoid dairy products for a while and see if your many years of skin problems, asthma, hay fever, iron deficiency, recurrent sinusitis and ear infections, or persistent obesity disappear like snow under a hot sun. You could reduce not only your weight but also your osteoporosis. I will come back to this.

MILK IS MADE FOR CALVES

Just like human milk is meant for babies, a cow's milk is meant for her calf. Not a single other mammal drinks milk into adulthood, and especially not milk from another mammal. You would find it weird to watch a mature horse drink from a cow's udders. Milk is created for newborn mammals. This is as nature has intended it, and there are good reasons for it. (Okay, with the possible exception of the occasional frothy cappuccino…) I'm not saying that *some* milk or dairy is really bad for you; the problem is that you're probably ingesting much too much.

Lactose Must Be Broken Down by Lactase

Milk contains lactose, also called milk sugars, which can be broken down only if the enzyme lactase is created in the small intestine. About 90 percent of adult Europeans and Americans make this enzyme, but if you're of Asian or African descent, chances are high that after infancy you no longer have this enzyme.

Lactose intolerance is not a disease.
Nature could never have imagined we would
wish to drink milk after babyhood.
Two out of three people worldwide are not
built for drinking milk after infancy.

Expensive Poo

Anyone who does not create this enzyme or doesn't create enough of it is labeled "lactose intolerant," which means that your intestines cannot digest milk. Instead it can cause abdominal pain, flatulence, cramps, diarrhea, and bloating. Over the longer term, that creates a sticky, mucous lining—a biofilm—on the inside of your small intestine, which limits the absorption of nutrients. No matter how healthily you eat, you will poop out most of the vitamins and minerals unused and your body will slowly but surely become malnourished. You can understand how, in the long term, this could cause all sorts of health problems. In addition, this attack on your intestinal wall can lead to a leaky gut, and you really don't want that. Read more about a leaky gut in Chapter 2.

Dairy and Gluten Are Allergens

Allergens are substances that people cannot deal with very well. Along with grains containing gluten, dairy is one of the food groups that most commonly lead to chronic inflammation, because a lot of people, often unnoticeably, do not tolerate and digest them well. Half of those sensitive to gluten are also sensitive to dairy. Chronic inflammation is the basis of many chronic diseases. Unfortunately, we women are more sensitive to chronic inflammation than men. Read more about this in Chapter 7.

More and more people are becoming allergic to or intolerant of certain foods. The annoying thing is that an intolerance is hard to measure. If a test shows that you aren't allergic to milk or milk products, it doesn't necessarily mean that you tolerate them very well.

Milk Is a Form of Sugar

If your gut doesn't create enough lactase, the milk sugar that arrives in your small intestine is converted into glucose and galactose, two forms of sugars that can be absorbed by your intestines. Everything that ends in ose is a form of sugar. Bingo: milk is also a form of sugar! There's a reason why people become addicted to milk, and just like sugar, it can be really fattening.

Milk Is Fattening, and That's as It Should Be

Sugar is fattening, and that is precisely its purpose: a calf puts on 250 kilos—that's 550 pounds!—in its first year thanks to its mother's milk sugars. Cow's milk also contains a growth hormone known as IGF-1. IGF stands for "insulin-like growth factor." You've already read how too much insulin in your body can make you fat. IGF-1 is a natural growth hormone intended for calves, not for you. Struggling with your weight and eating a lot of dairy products? Eliminate dairy and see what it does for you. You might be very surprised.

MILK HAS BECOME HIGHLY PROCESSED CHEMICAL FOOD

Please be aware that you can develop a lactose intolerance over the course of your life. Even if as a child or young woman you had no issues, that can suddenly change. If you're bloated or uncomfortable after using dairy, be warned. Rumbling intestines, stomach or abdominal pain, diarrhea, or constipation may also indicate a growing intolerance to milk products. This may have to do with your gut becoming more vulnerable, but it may also be because, worldwide, dairy cows are genetically doctored to make sure they're going to produce more milk. Our grandparents' cows gave two and a half gallons of milk a day. Dairy cows now produce 13 gallons. This is not as nature intended. The milk from these cows also contains a different type of protein (beta casein A1 instead of type A2), which is probably the cause of the current increase in lactose intolerance in Europe and North America, though there is still much uncertainty about that.

Milk Contains a Boost of Estrogens

Genetic tinkering of dairy cows is not the only problem. Nowadays cows get so much "power food" that they can be milked even while pregnant. Pregnant mammals make extremely high levels of estrogen to ensure, among other things, the growth of the fetus. These extremely high estrogen levels also end up in our milk—estrogens intended for a calf, not for us. Drinking that milk means a dose of foreign estrogens in your body.

In the dairy industry, the calf is usually taken away from the mother right after birth, and the cow immediately becomes stressed out. Cow's milk, therefore, also contains a lot of stress hormones. You then ingest these stress hormones by drinking milk or eating other forms of dairy. Naturally, this means that many dairy cows are not really healthy and strong. As happens regularly, if one has any disease, such as udder inflammation, antibiotics are immediately used. These are a hormone disruptor for your estrogen–progesterone balance and a threat to your healthy intestinal flora. Your milk contains estrogen, stress hormones, and antibiotics, and so do all the dairy products made from it. This is not something to be happy about. In the context of avoiding hormone-disrupting substances, it's worth seriously considering largely eliminating milk and milk products from your diet. Dairy is no longer the same product our grandparents consumed.

"Yes, but then what about my bones?" you might be thinking. We've all learned that calcium from milk will help to keep our bones strong.

WHOLE MILK, NOT SKIM

Do you, like me, enjoy the occasional frothy cappuccino? Then use organic whole milk for that. Organic milk contains less in the way of hormone disruptors, and the fat in whole milk helps your body to absorb the milk's minerals and vitamins more easily. Try goat milk or nondairy milk too, and remember to sprinkle a little cinnamon on top. Cinnamon is yummy, contains easily absorbable calcium, and helps keep your blood glucose level stable.

HOW DOES A COW GET HEALTHY BONES?

The dairy industry has fabricated a nice story: bones consist of calcium, milk contains calcium, so drink milk because it's good for your bones. It seems logical, but your body is much more complex than this simple equation. The Netherlands, where I live, is in the top five countries for dairy use and, at the same time, in the top five for oste-oporosis. Dozens of studies have now shown that milk is not good for bones. This is because there is a difference between calcium intake and calcium absorption. It turned out, from a 12-year investi-gation of 77,000 women aged 34 to 59, that women who drank more than two glasses of milk a day were 45 percent *more* likely to have fractures than women who drank only one glass a week.[1]

Calcium from Milk Is Hard to Absorb

Calcium from milk (calcium carbonate) is hard for your body to absorb. Calcium is readily absorbed by your blood only when cal-cium and magnesium occur in a of ratio of 2 to 1. Dairy contains too little magnesium, making this ratio 4 to 1. As a result, the acidity—the pH of your blood—decreases. So milk makes your blood acidic. To prevent this drop in pH, the acid is neutralized by calcium that's leeched from your bones and teeth! Your bones and teeth are the cal-cium storage supply used to regulate the pH of your blood. Cow's milk also contains phosphorus, which attaches itself to calcium, mak-ing it even harder to absorb.

So how do you take good care of your bones? A healthy cow has strong bones. Does she drink milk? No. She gets calcium from grass—vegetables, in other words. We can also get our calcium this way, because vegetables contain a form of calcium that is eas-ily digestible for our body. Good sources of calcium are all kinds of green vegetables and dried herbs, raw nuts and seeds, tempeh, and nettle tea. Plant-based milk made from raw nuts or seeds is also an excellent source of calcium. You'll find a recipe for homemade nut milk on page 8.

Vitamin D and Magnesium

To absorb calcium properly from the intestines, you need vitamin D. You get this from sunlight, so going outside every day is important. Unfortunately, if you live north of the 37th parallel in the northern hemisphere or south of it in the southern hemisphere—that's all the UK, all of Canada, states from Utah through Virginia and north, Tasmania, or south of Auckland—your latitude is too far from the equator to provide enough vitamin D from sunlight. Magnesium is another mineral that is important for healthy and strong bones. Many women have a magnesium deficiency, because you pee it out if you're under a lot of stress. Vitamin D and magnesium are, therefore, two vitamins that you should consider as a supplement. More on this in Chapter 12.

....

Dried mixed Provençal herbs are
valuable sources of calcium: basil, chervil, parsley,
oregano, and rosemary. Use plenty of them.

....

Physical Activity Is a Healthy Diet for Strong Bones

From the age of 35 on, we lose bone density. Women are affected more than men because bone loss is accelerated by the decline of the hormones progesterone and estrogen. Exercise is essential to keep your bones healthy and strong, so let them work for you. Training with weights, brisk walking, yoga, running, tennis, and dancing are all fine. Choose something you like, and keep doing it until you're 100!

Bone tissue is a remarkable, living substance that continues to develop through your whole life. It is continuously breaking itself down, but it also builds itself back up, as long as you continue to use your bones. By working out, you build up not only your bones but also your muscles. You need them both, no matter how old you get.

ARE YOU ADDICTED TO YOGURT OR CHEESE?

Every supermarket has a huge stock of dairy products waiting for you. I hope it is now clear to you that products like sweet yogurt drinks, pink cream cheese with strawberry flavoring, and pudding with fake rum and raisins are all very healthy for the dairy manufacturer's wallet but bad for your health. Don't be tempted by all these highly processed, addictive sweet foods.

Plain Yogurt

Even plain yogurt has some disadvantages. The main ingredient is milk, which contains quite a few substances that aren't healthy for you, as you've just read. Yogurt is cultured or fermented milk. Fermentation is a healthy process because lactose is broken down and healthy bacterial cultures arise, ones that make your gut flora happy. Unfortunately, the food industry uses easily processed bacterial cultures, because the yogurt should always taste the same, and they omit the necessary healthy yeasts because otherwise the packaging will bulge and explode.

Pasteurized yogurt no longer contains live acidophilus bacteria and ultimately has no healthy effect on your intestines. On the contrary—factory yogurt is a product that can contaminate your gut and intestinal flora. The levorotatory lactic acid in this yogurt is difficult to digest, and not all the lactose is broken down during fermentation. Do you like to eat yogurt every morning for breakfast? Just be aware that that is a missed opportunity for other nutrients that your body desperately needs. Variety is important, and there are so many other delicious and easy-to-make breakfasts.

....

Remember: if you almost panic when you realize you have to do without a certain food, it's probably doing something to you that's not healthy.

....

Addicted to Cheese?

I totally understand when you say you can't live without cheese. Cheese is something I myself occasionally eat because I find it so delicious. However, I've had clients who ate more than a pound of cheese a week, and that's not such a good idea. Apart from the milk sugars, there are two reasons why milk, yogurt, and cheese are addictive. If you find it difficult to eliminate them from your diet and you occasionally feel depressed or lethargic, this is important information.

Dairy Contains Exorphin

Exorphins are substances that, in our body, should be broken down by an enzyme. If this enzyme is not working properly or you eat too many exorphins, these exorphins take the place of your body's own endorphins, including dopamine and serotonin, the hormones that make you feel good. On top of that, exorphins not only deceive your endorphin system, but also affect the function of insulin, stress hormones, and your immune system.

Exorphins are found in gluten-containing grains, dairy products (the exorphin in dairy is called *casein*), soy, spinach, and certain fungi, but for the most part, soy, casein in dairy, and gluten in grains are the culprits.

Do you believe that yogurt helps against constipation? This doesn't mean it's healthy. Chances are high that your intestines struggle to digest it.

If you get a good feeling from eating exorphins (do you ever crave a cheese sandwich?), there's a good chance your body can't properly digest them. You might temporarily feel good, but then the feeling disappears, so you'll need to eat exorphins again to get the feeling back. The stronger the addiction, the more you need those exorphins, and the stronger your craving for cheese sandwiches.

The addictive power of exorphins may be stronger in women with estrogen dominance.

Dairy Contains Casomorphin

The type of exorphin in milk and cheese is called casein. As much as 80 percent of all the proteins in cow's milk consist of casein. Casein can be broken down into another amino acid, casomorphin, a nephew of morphine and heroin. Casomorphin in your body can cause morphine-like effects: first a peak where you feel good, followed by fatigue and even depressed feelings. Casomorphin is an addictive substance—it's also called "dairy crack." It's probably in milk to create a bond between mother and young. In nature, this bond is necessary because the survival of mammalian young depends on it.

....

Do you feel like you're addicted to bread, cheese, or both? Limit them for a while or stop eating them completely and see what this does for you. Don't be surprised if you have temporary withdrawal symptoms and strong cravings. Before long, you'll probably feel a lot more vital and more cheerful.

....

IS THERE A TIE BETWEEN ANIMAL PROTEIN AND CANCER?

Finally, I can't avoid this topic: many studies show a relationship between the overconsumption of animal protein and cancer. One well-known, extensive research study was done by scientist Colin Campbell. After years of tests on rats, he revealed he was able to turn cancer cells on and off by means of casein—milk protein. Dormant cancer cells in rats could be woken up by a high dose of casein. It seemed as if the clustering of cells (future tumors) even completely depended on the protein intake. On the other hand, rats that received a high dose of cancer-forming toxins, and that therefore had a great risk of cancer, could be protected from the toxins for a long time with a very low dose of animal protein. They didn't develop cancer. It seemed that an overdose of casein led to a growth of cancer cells because the action of the enzymes that protected rats against cancer was reduced. Naturally, Campbell also did tests with vegetable protein, but that produced no cancer growth. This research is described in detail in his book The China Study. Of course, research on rats doesn't necessarily apply to people.

But there have been other investigations, including with women. The Nurses' Health Study follows 88,000 subjects. Women who consumed a dairy product more than once a day were 44 percent more likely to have ovarian cancer than women who consumed hardly any dairy.[2] In dairy-rich societies, we have all learned that dairy is good for us. Eating plenty of dairy is good for the dairy industry's revenues, but not for my health or yours.

HEALTHY ALTERNATIVES TO DAIRY

Do you want to quit or cut down on dairy for a while to see what that does for your health and your weight? Good plan! Replace dairy with a mix of plant products and you'll feel like a new person after a few weeks. I've seen this happen often. If this is too radical for you, at least consider consuming less dairy from cows, especially milk, replacing it with goat's or sheep's milk. This dairy is easier for your intestines to digest because the protein structures match ours better. If you eat mostly vegetarian, this could be a good addition to your protein.

Choosing Dairy? Choose Organic and Whole Milk Products

If you do eat dairy, choose organic products as much as possible. Organic dairy has a different fermentation process, allowing more lactose to be broken down, which is kinder to your gut. Organic dairy also contains more of the healthy substance CLA (conjugated linoleic acid) and less in the way of hormone-disrupting substances.

Buy whole milk products, not skim, because the fats provide a better absorption of vitamins and minerals. You can easily make "milk" yourself from plant products such as nuts and seeds. With the help of kefir or other probiotics, you can also make a healthy form of yogurt that contains live lactic acid bacteria. See the recipe for coconut yogurt at the end of this chapter.

Choose Goat, Sheep, and Buffalo Cheese

Feta, ricotta, and sheep cheese are made from sheep's milk, and goat's cheese from goat's milk, of course. A good halloumi is made of a mix of sheep and goat cheese. A good mozzarella is made from buffalo milk, and Parmesan cheese is made from unpasteurized cow's cheese and is therefore healthier than cheese made from pasteurized milk. These are good alternatives if you do want to use some cheese. Ghee is the casein-free variation of butter, if you really want to avoid all casein. See Appendix A for more healthy alternatives.

Be Curious

You don't have to take anything from me—your body is always right. But if you don't feel as good as you could (and set the bar high!), then I recommend you reduce or drop dairy and see what that does for you. Be curious, try it out. Have the occasional tasty cappuccino if you want—I do—but drop all those other dairy products for a while. You'll be amazed at what it does for you. As a client of mine said when she was two weeks dairy-free, "Marjolein, my brain was foggy all those years! I never knew that my mind could be so clear!"

THE LIVING BACTERIA IN YOUR GUT

Kefir is made up of a group of live, naturally occurring, friendly bacteria and beneficial yeast. It looks like small heads of cauliflower. It contains probiotic cultures (lactic acid bacteria), and therefore falls into the category of probiotics. Probiotic bacteria survive the workings of your stomach acid and bile acids and arrive in your gut alive. Here they have a beneficial influence on your intestinal flora and the rest of your digestion, and thus on your overall health and appearance. You can consider using kefir as a natural dietary supplement after a course of antibiotics. You can also see it as a healthy option and have it every day. Water kefir and milk kefir are both available. Use water kefir to make delicious fresh drinks, and milk kefir to make yogurt.

....
Think of dairy as a treat, just like coffee
and alcohol. Enjoy it, but have it in moderation.
....

REMEMBER THIS

· Cow's milk is breast milk for calves—fine for calves but not for adult humans.
· Because of how cow's milk is produced, dairy products contain hormone-disrupting substances.
· Milk can affect the intestinal mucosa and ultimately lead to a leaky gut.
· The calcium in milk can't be easily absorbed by your bones. For healthy bones, you need vegetables and herbs, vitamin D, magnesium, and plenty of exercise.

- Dairy can make you fat; this is precisely the point of milk for a young mammal.
- Dairy contains substances to which your body can become addicted. They hinder the healthy function of your body's feel-good hormones.
- Some studies have demonstrated a relationship between excessive dairy consumption and cancer.
- There are plenty of healthy and delicious alternatives to dairy.

COCONUT YOGURT

Most yogurt sold in supermarkets doesn't contain live probiotics. For your gut, therefore, it's better to eat homemade yogurt. After much experimenting, I came up with this delicious coconut yogurt.

This is heavier than regular yogurt, so serve it like a dollop of whipped cream over fresh fruit or use it in desserts or smoothies. It's deliciously tangy like yogurt, but the texture is a bit grainier. You might need to just get used to that.

Use a squeaky-clean canning jar with a rubber ring that you can close tightly. Rinse the jar with hot water before use.

Here's What You Need
1 package (7 ounces) organic creamed coconut, without additives

2 probiotic capsules, about 1 billion (1 x 10^9) CFUs each

a 1½ pint canning jar

Here's How You Make It
Remove the creamed coconut from the package, put it in a small pot, and pour 1½ cups boiling water over it. Let soak about 15 minutes. The creamed coconut will be largely melted. Whisk the mixture until it's smooth. Allow it to cool to lukewarm. Open the two capsules of probiotics and pour the contents into the creamed coconut mix. Throw the capsules away. Stir well. Put the mixture in the canning jar, seal, and leave in a warm place in the house, such as a kitchen cupboard, for 24 hours. Above room temperature is fine. Shake the jar occasionally but don't open it yet.

After 24 hours, put the jar in the refrigerator; only now will the yogurt stiffen. After another 24 hours, it will be ready. Use caution when opening it, as the contents may have become pressurized. If you keep it in the fridge, the yogurt has about a 5-day shelf life.

A note on creamed coconut: If you can't get cubed creamed coconut, use the thick layer of cream at the top of an unshaken can of coconut milk.

POINT 6: INTESTINES DO NOT LIKE GLUTEN

FOR 20 YEARS I suffered from a lot of abdominal pain, bloating, constipation alternating with diarrhea, nausea, and unexplained mood swings and I was often very tired. I was tested for everything, but nothing ever showed up. Around my 40th birthday, my symptoms grew worse. By listening carefully to my body and paying attention to what I ate, I discovered that if I ate little or no bread, the symptoms stayed away. When I stopped eating bread (every now and then I have a slice because I still find it very tasty!), the symptoms did not return, and I suddenly lost 11 pounds. I now know that I'm sensitive to gluten.

I am convinced that many women who struggle with health problems (including persistent obesity) would do well to eliminate gluten for a while. I have seen miracles happen in women who have decided to avoid gluten for a time. The results were more than sufficient motivation for them to consume it very sparingly in future.

WHAT IS GLUTEN, ANYWAY?

Cereals contain proteins that we call gluten. The gluten protein gliadin in particular is a hard protein for your intestines to digest. Gluten is found in seven types of cereal: wheat, rye, barley, spelt, kamut, bulgur, and couscous. Couscous and bulgur are grain products made from wheat. Wheat contains the most aggressive form of the protein. Oats also contain a gluten protein—avenine—but this is the mildest form. Rice and corn are other cereals with mild gluten.

Gluten Is Allergenic

Along with dairy, gluten is at the top of the list of allergens: substances that a growing number of people do not tolerate well or to which they have allergic reactions. Most intestines are not happy with gluten.

Humans do not have the right enzymes to break down gluten into molecules small enough to easily digest. Undigested gluten in your gut is fantastic food for bad gut bacteria, fungi, and other organisms that can cause all kinds of abdominal and digestive complaints. Gluten can also damage your intestinal wall and result in a leaky gut. This will allow unwanted substances to enter your body via your blood, which in turn will lead to an immediate response by your immune system because the gluten doesn't belong there. A leaky gut is usually the beginning of a wide range of complaints and chronic diseases, including autoimmune disorders, conditions that affect women more men. You can read more about leaky gut in Chapter 2.

Celiac Disease

Celiac disease is an autoimmune disease. In celiac disease, the intestinal wall is severely damaged by undigested gluten. A doctor can determine if you have celiac disease or not, but a negative outcome (no celiac disease) does not mean that your intestines handle gluten well. You can have a form of gluten sensitivity that would not be flagged by most medical examinations. Celiac disease is black or white: either you have it or you don't. But there's a big gray area; that's what we call gluten sensitivity. Your gut can also be quite sensitive to gluten without you realizing it. I've lived with it for 20 years. Just like dairy, gluten causes a sensitivity that slowly sneaks into your life. For years you've eaten stacks of sandwiches, then suddenly you have issues. Of course it doesn't occur to you that those sandwiches (plus pasta, granola, toast, crackers, muffins, cakes, power bars, soups, sauces, and all those other processed products that contain wheat) could be the cause of the problem!

SYMPTOMS ARE YOUR BEST FRIENDS

Mild symptoms are your best friends: they tell you that something is out of balance and that it would be wise to investigate what could be going on with a curious and open mind. Even if you're symptom-free, take a look at how much gluten you ingest, even in the form of brown bread, which many still see as the basis of a healthy breakfast or lunch. I don't see it that way at all anymore.

OSTEOARTHRITIS IS MY BEST FRIEND

From her 40th birthday on, my mother, like her mother before her, suffered from arthritis in her fingers. The joints were thicker, and she had a lot of pain. I remember the many nights she sat in front of the TV in white gloves to let the ointment that she had rubbed on her fingers soak in. It didn't help—her fingers curved and became painful. For me it started around my 45th: a nagging throbbing in some joints and pain when bending them. It was during a vacation, when I don't always want to be smarter than sugar. Once I was home again, it receded. I made the link to my nutrition and found out that the sugars and the little gluten that I occasionally ate were the culprits. Now I know that I should pay close attention when that feeling in my fingers starts again, and that I then must eliminate sugars, alcohol, and gluten and provide my body with plenty of nutrients, mainly from vegetables. That has worked fine so far—over 10 years later, I have no problems. I now know that osteoarthritis is a signal of hidden inflammation. Pain in my finger joints is the weak spot where this hidden inflammation lets itself be known.

CEREALS ARE GRASSES

Humans have eaten cereals for only about 15,000 years. Just as lions don't nibble grass or zebras gnaw on gazelles, we humans were not built for cereals. But we began to eat them anyway.

Grains Aren't Easy to Eat

Pick an apple from the tree and you can eat it right away. You have to wash a carrot, but it's also immediately edible. Grains are essentially grasses, and almost all cereals must be processed before they are edible for us. The grains have to be separated from the stem and the husk removed from every grain; then the grains are finely ground, some water and yeast added, and the dough should be kneaded for a good while afterward. Then it needs to rise for hours and be baked in a hot oven. Only once it has cooled do we have something that we humans can eat. You probably wouldn't eat bread if you had to do all of this for yourself. In prehistoric times people did not eat grains. And our health did not improve when we began to do so.

Long Life but Bad Health

In his book *The Paleo Diet*, Remko Kuipers states that evolution is not about healthy aging but about producing many offspring.[1] In that sense, the invention of agriculture was a great success: farmers had more children. It was less successful in other senses, especially in the area of health. After extensive research, the American anthropologist and archaeologist Mark Nathan Cohen concluded, in *The Food Crisis in Prehistory*, that the introduction of agriculture worldwide was followed by an increase in growth disorders, malnutrition, and tooth decay. For overall human health, the introduction of agriculture was not so healthy. Many studies have now confirmed this.

WHEAT HAS BEEN GIVEN EXTRA STICKINESS

That wheat can't be digested very well by humans to begin with may not be the biggest problem. There is other food, after all, that requires some work before we put our teeth into it, such as meat or fish. The real problem is that in recent decades, wheat has been considerably doctored. The gluten in grains works like a kind of wallpaper paste: it keeps the substance of a dough together. For bakers this is a handy feature, because you can make thin pizza crusts, croissants, waffles, and whoppers of muffins, only with the stickiness of that paste. To even better accommodate bakers, new wheat strains have been developed, through hybridization and crossbreeding—strains that contain more gluten. These modern wheat strains would not even survive in nature: they need fertilizers and pesticides to make it. In other words, today's wheat products are very different from those of our grandparents.

Sharp Stones in Your Gut

That larger amount of gluten is fine for bakers, but not for your intestines, because it is precisely this gluten with extra adhesive force that is aggressive and even less digestible for your intestines. If your gut looks like a bicycle tire, then gluten is a gravel road with sharp stones. That can go well for a while, but you run the risk of getting a flat tire sooner or later. People who do not do well with wheat bread may, however, still respond well to spelt or rye bread: spelt and rye don't contain the aggressive type of gluten that wheat does. Now you also understand why spelt bread falls apart more easily than wheat bread. You definitely can't bake croissants with 100 percent spelt dough.

Wheat Proteins Have Changed, a Lot

In his book *Wheat Belly*, Dr. William Davis, a cardiologist specializing in preventive health care, expands on the hybridization of wheat and raises the question of whether the properties of our current wheat are still compatible with human health. Over the past decades, no one questioned whether all the new wheat strains could be tolerated by our digestive system. Davis writes that small changes in the structure of wheat proteins could be the difference between a destructive immune reaction in our body and no immune response at all. According to him, wheat proteins in particular have undergone substantial changes through hybridization.

....

Sugars, dairy, and grains are all addictive substances.

....

ADDICTION: THE THREE PARTNERS IN CRIME

Sugar, dairy, and cereals. I call them "the three partners in crime": all three are highly addictive substances. If you have a small panic attack at the very idea that you should eat less bread because it's not healthy for you, then it may be that your body is addicted—please be warned. I also struggled with this, despite the symptoms I experienced from eating bread, and I still have to be careful when I eat a small piece of bread. There's a strong temptation to eat more of it than that one little bit: I still find bread with a crisp crust incredibly tasty. Dr. William Davis writes about this in *Wheat Belly*: "So this is your brain on wheat: Digestion yields morphine-like compounds that bind to the brain's opiate receptors. It induces a form of reward, a mild euphoria. When the effect is blocked or no exorphin-yielding foods are consumed, some people can experience a distinctly unpleasant withdrawal."[2]

Cereals Are Sugar for
Your Blood Glucose Level

There is another correlation between sugar, dairy, and cereals: not only are they all addictive, but all three increase your blood glucose levels. If one thing is important for your hormone balance, it's a stable blood sugar level. Grains and dairy give your blood sugar a similar spike as sugar.

The system that ranks foods based on how fast your blood glucose level rises is called glycemic index (GI). The higher the GI, the more your blood glucose level is shifted out of balance. White table sugar has a GI of around 60. Did you know that a white dinner roll has a GI of about 90? Even a whole wheat roll has a GI of around 70, so it is not just the refined carbohydrates that are problematic. A brown bun or whole wheat sandwich has a similar effect on your blood glucose level as sugar. If you have something sweet on it, the effect is even greater. Be honest: a slice of bread with chocolate spread or jam is still basically just a pastry, isn't it? If you get hungry again an hour after eating a sandwich, then you now know why. The sandwich is triggering a similar blood sugar spike in your body as sweet foods do. Soon after that, a dip always follows, causing your body's survival instinct to kick in, clamoring for quick energy in the form of food that can give you a boost. You experience this as insatiable hunger or cravings that are hard to resist with willpower.

....

Did you think pumpernickel bread is healthy because it's such a nice dark brown? Malt bread gets its dark color from molasses, a form of sugar.

....

A World of Sugar Peaks

What is a pity in the West is that we're used to eating grains and milk, both when we get up and at noon, and to drinking large amounts of coffee or black tea. As a result, our blood glucose level keeps peaking. It's no wonder we need midmorning and midafternoon snacks: these are the times when our blood sugar level dips. It's no wonder type 2 diabetes, the result of fluctuating blood glucose levels and of insulin that has to take action, claims thousands of new victims every week.

CEREALS, SUGAR, DAIRY, AND YOUR BRAIN

Women are more affected than men by dementia. This used to be a brain disease that occurred only in older women, but just as with diabetes, we now see more younger women being affected, even in their 40s. In the film *Still Alice*, actress Julianne Moore impressively shows us how it looks when a woman in the prime of her life is affected by Alzheimer's disease, a form of dementia. How can so many young women now be affected by this "old age" disease?

Type 3 Diabetes

In 2005, scientific articles described Alzheimer's disease as a new form of diabetes. It's now also called type 3 diabetes. People with type 2 diabetes are four times more likely than others to get Alzheimer's. The cause is similar. Type 2 diabetes is largely a result of the pancreas having to produce insulin again and again to lower the blood sugar level. If this happens too often, cells become deaf to this insulin; this is "insulin resistance." Eventually your pancreas becomes exhausted from producing the extra insulin, and this is referred to as type 2 diabetes. You need to artificially get your blood glucose level back down with the help of medications or injected insulin.

Inflammation Is Poison to Your Cells

As with type 2 diabetes, the underlying cause of Alzheimer's begins with consumption of things (especially sugars and bad carbohydrates) that increase your blood glucose level. Frequent and prolonged high blood glucose levels lead to inflammation in your body, and this inflammation eventually reaches your brain. You can think of inflammation as poison for your cells, including your brain cells. In 2014, American neurologist Dr. David Perlmutter published

Grain Brain. In this book, Perlmutter describes the danger of sugars, carbohydrates, and grains, because they form the basis for chronic inflammation, and he explains the link between chronic inflammation and neurodegenerative diseases including Alzheimer's, other forms of dementia, and Parkinson's.

He writes, "Remember, at the heart of virtually every disorder and disease is inflammation. When we introduce anything to the body that triggers an inflammatory response, we set ourselves up for taking on much greater risk for a medley of health challenges, from chronic daily nuisances like headaches and brain fog to severe ailments such as depression and Alzheimer's. We can even make a case for linking gluten sensitivity with some of the most mysterious brain diseases that have eluded doctors for millennia, such as schizophrenia, epilepsy, depression, bipolar disorder, and, more recently, autism and ADHD."[3]

Dr. Perlmutter is convinced that brain diseases can be reversed through nutrition and lifestyle changes. He recommends eliminating sugars, carbohydrates, and gluten and choosing healthy fats. A healthy brain needs plenty of healthy fats to function properly; your brain is 60 percent fat. He, as a doctor, has come to understand that cholesterol plays a vital role in the functioning of the brain, and he highlights the fact that the use of statins is probably a cause of many brain diseases.

Statins are medications used to lower cholesterol. In 2012, a study of more than 160,000 postmenopausal women showed that the use of statins increased the risk of diabetes by 71 percent.[4]

Statins Probably Increase the Risk of Alzheimer's

In 2009, a report by MIT's Stephanie Seneff suggested that statins in combination with a low-fat diet are likely a cause of Alzheimer's disease. She explains that problems result in the brain because statins sabotage the liver's ability to produce cholesterol. Cholesterol is essential for a healthy brain.[5] Now more and more doctors and researchers concur with this view.

If you use statins, dig into this issue and consult your doctor about the best way to taper off. Eating following the points of the Nutrition Compass can definitely help you.

DON'T RUN STRAIGHT TO THE GLUTEN-FREE AISLE!

The gluten-free market is growing by about 33 percent every year. More and more people want or need to eat gluten-free, and the marketing campaigns of producers of gluten-free products are helping to show them that road. However, I advise you to avoid the gluten-free section in the supermarket. Many of the products, including gluten-free bread, contain all kinds of sugars that imitate the stickiness of gluten. Gluten is often replaced by sugars or unhealthy fats. Most of the products are merely good examples of artful tinkering, so read the labels. On top of that, they're very expensive. It would be better to spend this money on healthier gluten-free products that you can easily make yourself and that are much tastier.

If you don't have celiac disease, it's not necessary to eat 100 percent gluten-free. If you eliminate most of your bread and crackers and all types of cakes, sweets, and other pastries plus pasta made from wheat, you're already a long way to a better diet. Delicious gluten-free pasta made from quinoa, buckwheat, and seaweed is available, and you can easily make your own granola with rolled oats as a base. Pick up gluten-free crackers, and make pancakes with gluten-free flours, such as buckwheat. See Appendix A for more healthy alternatives.

Choose 100 Percent Spelt Sourdough Bread

If you occasionally want to eat bread, choose the best quality you can get. Sourdough bread has a lot of advantages. It's much better for your intestines than yeast bread, because it's fermented. Spelt bread is better than wheat. This makes sourdough spelt bread a good choice if you still want to eat bread. Sweet potato bread is also a good choice. Baking your own bread is, of course, the best!

If you no longer eat food from packages, bags, and mixes, you automatically consume much less of the wheat hidden in creamy soups, sauces, meats, and prepackaged or frozen meals. You cannot imagine the crazy things to which the food industry adds wheat! Then there's the wheat hidden in your cosmetics and lipstick. (Yes, really! Because of the stickiness of gluten.) You just have to take wheat's presence for granted... unless, of course, you have celiac disease.

If you do drastically reduce the amount of bread in your diet, be prepared for withdrawal symptoms such as fatigue, brain fog, mood swings, and cravings for carbohydrates or sweets. This should fade after a few days. Drink plenty of water to dispose of the waste products. Just persevere, because you will become much healthier in return.

·······································

Bread needs only flour, water, yeast or sourdough, and some salt. All other ingredients are a strain on your body. Bread can be called "spelt bread" even if it's only 1 percent spelt and 99 percent wheat, so read labels!

·······································

REMEMBER THIS

- Certain cereals contain gluten, a substance that does not get on well with your intestines. Undigested gluten can cause many health concerns. Wheat contains the most aggressive form of gluten.
- Because of the hybridization of wheat varieties, today's strains of wheat contain a lot more gluten than 50 years ago. The food industry hides wheat in many products.
- You can over time develop a sensitivity to gluten. This does not always show up in test results, and health complaints are often not linked to gluten sensitivity.

- Grains, just like sugars and dairy, are heavily addictive substances.
- Grains have the same effect on your body as sugars. Constantly having a high blood glucose level is related not only to type 2 diabetes, but also to brain diseases such as dementia, because of the inflammatory reactions that it triggers.
- It can do you good to eliminate, or at least strictly limit, bread, especially wheat bread, from your diet. If you do eat bread, choose the best quality that you can get.

PROVENÇAL VEGETABLE BREAD

By now you have understood that I try to hide vegetables and herbs in everything I can—even in bread. Sometimes I long to eat something breadlike. Even though I've pretty much kicked my bread habit, I always have a few slices of this vegetable bread in the freezer. You can use all sorts of different vegetables as long as the harder vegetables are chopped very fine. It's especially good to vary the herbs, and try replacing the tomatoes with olives.

You can easily make almond flour yourself in a good blender. That makes it cheap and less perishable.

Here's What You Need
½ cup brown rice flour
½ cup almond flour
1 red onion, very finely chopped
2 cloves garlic, finely chopped
1 cup grated zucchini
1 cup grated carrot
½ cup finely chopped sun-dried tomatoes
3 tablespoons mixed Provençal herbs
a few pinches of Celtic Sea salt
a few turns of fresh pepper
1 teaspoon baking soda (sodium bicarbonate)
4 large eggs
1 tablespoon coconut oil
1 tablespoon lemon juice

Here's How You Make It
Preheat the oven to 350°F. Put the rice and almond flours in a large bowl. Add the chopped onion, garlic, zucchini, carrot, sun-dried tomatoes, herbs, salt, pepper, and baking soda. Stir well. Beat the

eggs in a mixer until frothy. Add the eggs and coconut oil to the vegetable–nut mixture. Finally, add the lemon juice. Mix well.

Line the long sides of a loaf pan with parchment paper or grease the pan, and put the mix in the pan. Use a spatula to make a slit lengthwise down the middle. Cover the pan with aluminum foil and bake for about 20 minutes in the oven. Remove the foil after 20 minutes and bake another 20 minutes. Remove from the pan and let it completely cool on a wire rack before slicing it.

12

POINT 7: EAT MANY DIFFERENT THINGS (BUT DON'T EAT TOO MUCH)

A FEW YEARS AGO, my sisters and I had to clean out our parents' house. At the back of a large oak cupboard we found the dishes my parents had bought in the first years of their marriage for Sundays and holidays. I was sure that I held the stack of breakfast plates, but to my surprise my sister took out a stack of plates that were even smaller. There weren't any other plates. We drew the conclusion that the smallest plates had to be the breakfast plates and the slightly larger ones the dinner plates. We were amazed at the size of them: they were so small! At that moment, I realized that we have been eating off progressively larger plates and that, probably unnoticed, the portions that we eat have also become larger.

BE THE BOSS OF YOUR STOMACH

There used to be only 6.5-ounce bottles of cola; now there are 26-ounce bottles. Bags of chips and candy are offered in ever larger "family" packs, while the size of our families has declined. In many restaurants, the portions are bigger than ever, and all-you-can-eat buffets are popular. Make a fist and look at it: what you see is the normal size of your stomach. Now you know how much you can eat if you want to fill 80 percent of your stomach. If 80 percent of your stomach is filled, you should *feel* full. For many people that normal feeling of satiety has been kidnapped by the food industry and all its addictive products, accompanied by a lack of nutrients that our body needs. That is why it is so important to avoid synthetically crafted processed foods as much possible and to eat real, unprocessed food. Then a natural sense of satiety will return.

Even if you eat "real" healthy food, it's wise to not fill more than 80 percent of your stomach. If you eat so much that your stomach is totally full, really 100 percent, your body will produce insulin. By now you know the disadvantages of excessive insulin production.

Eat Slowly and with Attention

How you eat is perhaps just as important as what you eat. It takes 20 minutes before your stomach sends a signal to your brain that it is full. That is why it's important to eat slowly and with full attention. Let your ears, nose, and eyes enjoy the food; eat with all your senses.

Are you a fast eater? That's a habit that you once learned and therefore can unlearn. Put your cutlery down after each bite and grab it again only after your mouth is empty. An additional advantage is that you are probably chewing better, making digestion begin in your mouth. Your stomach and intestines won't need to work as hard and will be able to focus on other important tasks such as creating enough stomach acid or producing serotonin, which makes you feel good. Ideally, don't drink with a meal; it dilutes your gastric juices.

Forget What You Knew about Quantities

If you eat more real food, you'll notice that you can eat quite a lot. Several of the women I've mentored had to eat more than they were accustomed to in order not to lose too much weight. No, this is not a sales pitch! If you start to replace sweets, dairy, and cereals with a lot of vegetables, herbs, fruits, nuts, and seeds, you'll be amazed by how much you can eat without gaining weight. However, I also know women who came to realize that they actually had been eating quite a lot and no longer needed as much.

If your diet changes, release old patterns and ideas about the quantities of food you need. Take the time to eat, and be aware of when you've had enough. With age, sooner or later your metabolism will slow down, which means that your body will gradually need less food. Don't just eat out of habit, but eat mindfully, so that not only your stomach but all the cells in your body will be nourished. The only scientifically proven method to slow down the aging process is to limit the intake of food. Apparently our body "wears out" faster if we keep giving it a lot of food.

....

If you replace the quantity in your diet with quality, chances are you'll need less food than you were used to eating.

....

EAT AS MUCH VARIETY AS POSSIBLE

No food is completely good or completely bad; good or bad depends on quantity. Water is healthy, but if you drink more than two and a half gallons (10 liters) of water a day, it can kill you. This applies to all healthy products. The other way around, something that might not be as healthy we may still need in small amounts. A little nitrate keeps your blood pressure at a healthy level; you need a little phytic acid to bind to toxins in your body; and free radicals in your body also have a function. So it's a good idea to ensure the greatest possible variety: eat a lot of things in small quantities.

TWO-THIRDS OF THE SUPERMARKET CONSISTS OF THREE CROPS

In his book *In Defense of Food*, Michael Pollan shows us how poor the variety of our diet is. Historically, humankind has eaten about 80,000 different crops, of which about 3,000 are used all over the world. Pollan looked at the current US eating patterns and came to the conclusion that of the average daily consumption of calories, 23 percent consisted of corn, 10 percent of soy, and no less than 32 percent of wheat. Sixty-five percent of what Americans eat consists of just three crops: wheat, corn, and soy.[1] Do the rest of us, including my fellow Europeans, do much better?

....

From the moment you eliminate junk food and store-bought processed food, you automatically have a much more varied diet, because more one-sided than *that* is hardly possible!

....

Give Your Body Many Nutrients

So don't eat too much, but do eat the widest possible variety of foods. Any unprocessed food product has its own nutritional value for you. It would be nice if you got a text message in the morning from your body saying something like, "Good morning! Today would you be sure to have an extra dose of vitamin C, magnesium and chromium, a bit of theobromine, and a helping of anthocyanins?" Unfortunately, this doesn't happen. The best tactic is to give your body as much variety as possible so that it gets a large amount of nutrients to be able to get to work.

Choose a Colorful Palette for Your Plate

Vegetables are an important part of the Nutrition Compass. It is advisable to strive for over a pound (500 grams) of vegetables per day. That's a lot, I'll admit. It's best if they are spread throughout the day. Fortunately, there's a lot to choose from. In the Netherlands alone, there are more than 70 types of vegetables available any day. What a luxury! In any season, you can give different vegetables the starring role. At one of my workshops it became apparent that most women use the same 10 vegetables. So most women still have about 60 new vegetables to discover! How many different vegetables do you use? Mushrooms, by the way, are officially not considered vegetables but are definitely a valuable addition. All vegetables have their own colors, and it turns out that each color contains a separate nutrient for your body. Choose variety and make sure you ingest different-colored vegetables every day. Salads are, of course, fantastic for a wide variety of colors.

ADD SUPERFOODS AS SUPPLEMENTS

Superfoods are a valuable addition when it comes to variety. Superfoods are natural, often unprocessed plant foods such as seeds, dried berries, algae, or fats that have a naturally high concentration of nutritional value. Often they come from areas where Indigenous people have known for centuries that these foods will give you a boost of energy, health, and stamina.

Let me stress first that fresh vegetables, herbs, fruits, and sprouts are the very best superfoods that nature gives us—the fresher the better. So the closer these are grown to your home, the better it is. I see other superfoods as a complement to and variation on this sound basis. In this case, also choose the best quality you can find. And just as you don't eat broccoli every day, it's good to vary superfoods and not eat the same ones every day. They can have a powerful effect.

Superfoods Are Not Healthy by Definition

Superfoods have been discredited because some of them (such as goji berries) were found to be sprayed with significant amounts of pesticides. If the demand for certain products increases, in the short term there will always be producers that try to take advantage to profit financially. Dried cranberries are also seen as superfoods but are often covered with a thick layer of sugar syrup, because they are naturally very sour. The label "superfoods" does not by definition mean that a food is healthy.

My Favorite Superfoods

Superfoods that I use regularly are hempseed, chia seed, goji berries, flaxseed, bee pollen, raw cacao, spirulina, chlorella, and maca. In smoothies I also use mixes of greens, such as wheatgrass powder and barley grass powder.

BETTER HORMONE BALANCE WITH MACA?

Maca has been used for thousands of years as a power source and medicine by the local population where it is grown, high in the Andes. Incan messengers, who often had to walk for days, were given maca. Maca was also known to improve memory, fight depression, and increase libido. The special feature of maca is that it affects your hormones as a so-called adaptogen. An adaptogen is a substance that encourages the body toward improvement and a better balance in its production of our hormones. During menopause, maca can stimulate our endocrine system to restore hormone balance as much as possible. In contrast to other plant products, such as soy, black cohosh, and flaxseed, maca contains no plant hormones or phytoestrogens, so it has no effect on the hormone glands, which in time could become lazy if too many hormone substances are ingested. So with maca the body will produce the appropriate hormones, depending on what it needs. You'll have to try maca to see if it works for you. Women's experiences vary; for some it has an obvious benefit, for others not.

See superfoods as a complement to a healthy diet. Adding expensive superfoods to highly processed commercial foods or junk food meals makes no sense. Besides, what counts as expensive? Ten dollars for a bag of high-protein, nutritious hempseed, or one dollar for a can of tomato soup? If you look at the effects it will have in your body, then *any* amount for the can of tomato soup is too high: it will cost you your health.

ADD NUTRITIONAL SUPPLEMENTS

Dr. Christiane Northrup, a women's doctor and author of *Women's Bodies, Women's Wisdom*, writes that she considers supplementation as nutrition in itself.[2] I agree with her. Let's adopt her opinion.

Supplements Aren't Magic Pills

Does taking supplements make you think of taking medications? Many women make this association and are therefore not in favor of them. However, over the past 50 years, thousands of studies have shown that nutritional supplements can protect you against a wide range of conditions. But just like good nutrition, you need to use them for years; supplements aren't magic pills that can rid you of your symptoms in just a few days. As described in Chapter 3, chances are high that you don't consume enough nutrients. You can eat only a certain amount of food and thus nutrients every day. At some point you're full. Using supplements is the only way to get enough nutrients. The risk of ingesting too few nutrients is many times greater than that of ingesting too many.

Recommended Daily Amount:
To Just Not Die

The recommended dietary allowance (RDA) is the quantity of a nutrient that a national health organization recommends the average person ingest daily. Governments started setting out these recommendations in the 1930s and 1940s. Their purpose was to avoid diseases such as scurvy or beriberi. They were intended to prevent you from dying. In light of the arrival of all our modern stress and toxins and the erosion of nutrients in our diet, it's logical to expect that these quantities would have been increased considerably over the past 85 years. However, oddly enough, that's not the case.

Orthomolecular Supplementation:
To Age Full of Health and Vitality

The term *orthomolecular medicine* was first used in 1968 by two-time Nobel Prize winner Linus Pauling. Pauling suggested that the optimal daily amount of vitamins and minerals we need nowadays is much larger than we can get from our normal diet, no matter how healthily we eat. The amounts of minerals, vitamins, and other nutrients that orthomolecular medicine recommends for us is much higher than government recommendations. Orthomolecular medicine is aimed at helping people age as full of vitality and health as possible, a target that I find a lot better than mere survival.

HOW MUCH VITAMIN D IS ENOUGH?

In 2011, 40 top international vitamin D researchers joined together in a "Call to D*Action," advising widespread vitamin D testing. Recommended dietary vitamin D intake in the United States at the time was just 600 IU (15 mcg) a day. But the researchers noted that "40–75% of the world's population is vitamin D deficient," and that "even in southern [US] climates, 55% of African Americans and 22% of Caucasians are deficient." They recommended "that everyone have their vitamin D level tested and make sure it is between 100–150 nmol/L," a level that for many people would require many times higher vitamin D intake: "The latest Institute of Medicine (IOM) report, 2010, indicates 10,000 IU/day is considered the NOAEL (no observed adverse effect level). 4,000 IU/day can be considered a safe upper intake level for adults aged 19 and older."[3]

When It Comes to Supplements, Cheap Is Expensive

It can be a challenge to find good food supplements. Anyone can put supplements on the market, and many dietary supplements consist of synthetic materials. The best supplements are based on natural substances and not synthetic ones. The latter can even be harmful, because if your body can't properly eliminate them, they can accumulate in your blood. Fish oil can be contaminated with mercury or may already be oxidized before it's put in capsules and on the market. This will not make you healthier. So choose renowned orthomolecular brands, and be aware that cheap usually means expensive when it comes to supplements.

Supplements can never replace real food. It's not for nothing that you often must take them with a meal: the substances in your food supplement often need other substances from your diet to be effective.

Know What You Swallow

Nutritional supplementation is hyped and has thus become a chaotic jungle. Many women randomly buy supplements that they actually get nothing from. At best, their health isn't damaged. Research on supplements often focuses only on the effects of one particular supplement, not a whole cocktail of supplements. We don't really know how a cocktail of supplements will affect the body, so be very cautious.

Inform Yourself Well and Seek Professional Help

It's important to become well informed about supplementation. If you want to use more than the basic supplements listed below, consult a good orthomolecular physician or therapist who can test for what you really need. If you take medications, are pregnant, or are not completely healthy and you want to use supplements, talk with your doctor or nutritionist. Supplements can sometimes get in the way of drugs.

....

For maintaining a healthy weight, it can
be important to use a good
multivitamin and mineral supplement.

....

MULTIVITAMINS: GOOD FOR CARDIOVASCULAR HEALTH AND A HEALTHY WEIGHT

Most women die of cardiovascular diseases. By 2009, however, research had shown that women who took multivitamins for a decade were 28 percent less likely to die from cardiovascular disease. Moreover, the cells of these female multivitamin users were biologically younger than those of the control group. This was measured by looking at the telomeres (an indicator of the aging process) and the quality of the DNA. As if this were not enough, another study, of overweight Chinese women, showed that those who took a multivitamin lost measurably more weight than the placebo group.[4]

BASIC SUPPLEMENTATION FOR WOMEN

What supplements can be considered basic, which ones are good for you to take every day? The recommendations below were established after consultation with gynecologist and orthomolecular physician Barbara Havenith.

A Good Multivitamin and Mineral Supplement

Start with an orthomolecular multivitamin and mineral preparation (also known as a "multi"). This is a mix of various vitamins and minerals. Vitamins and minerals work together and have several tasks in your body. For every task they need some other partner vitamin or mineral. In a good orthomolecular multi, these will be present in the right proportions. If you're afraid of osteoporosis, you shouldn't take only calcium, because calcium needs magnesium and vitamin D to be effective. Taking calcium-only tablets makes no sense. By using a good quality multivitamin and mineral supplement, you get a wide variety of vitamins and minerals that can work together. Spirulina is considered a 100 percent natural "multi" due to the large variety of nutrients in it.

Vitamin C: Your Best Friend during Stress

Almost all mammals make their own vitamin C during times of illness or stress. Humans lost this ability somewhere during our evolution. That's too bad, because we're surrounded by more causes of stress than many other mammals. When you consider that the toxic substances in your body are only a small portion of your stress, you'll agree that it's a good idea to take at least 1,000 mg vitamin C a day. If you're under a lot of stress, a higher dosage, such as 3,000 mg, is recommended. Take this distributed throughout the day.

VITAMIN C HELPS AGAINST MANY CONDITIONS

Over dozens of years, many scientific studies have been conducted on the use of (high doses of) vitamin C. Over 30 diseases and conditions have been established against which intake of vitamin C had a positive effect. These range from high blood pressure to eye problems and from Alzheimer's to cardiovascular disease.

Do you often suffer from bladder infections? Vitamin C makes your urine acidic, so that the problem bacteria can't survive. Take extra vitamin C for a while. And if you feel a cold or flu coming on, you can temporarily take more vitamin C each day.

Some superfoods are high in vitamin C, such as camu camu, acai berries, and acerola berries. These are natural sources of vitamin C and are also available in powder or tablets.

SUPPORT YOUR ADRENAL GLANDS WITH VITAMIN C

Your adrenal glands use more vitamin C than any other tissue, because they need ascorbic acid (vitamin C) to produce the stress hormones cortisol and adrenaline. Too much stress exhausts your adrenal glands, because, among other things, they have inadequate vitamin C. So make sure you get enough vitamin C, especially when under stress.

Vitamin D: Protection against (Breast) Cancer

Vitamin D is not actually a vitamin but a hormone that was developed very early in our evolution. As a result, it has many functions in our body and a lack of it can lead to a wide range of problems. We can create Vitamin D in our skin when we are exposed to sunlight. Unfortunately, many of us live too far from the equator to make enough vitamin D, even in the summer. That's annoying because it's not easy to get enough of this vitamin from our food. It's found mainly in oily fish.

BONES NEED VITAMIN D

One in four women over the age of 55 suffers from osteoporosis. Menopause accelerates the process of bone loss because our estrogen production decreases. Luckily, bones are a living substance and you can reverse this process. For strong bones, you need vitamin D. You also need enough protein, calcium, magnesium, and vitamin K, and plenty of physical activity.

....

Do you suffer from osteoarthritis or arthritis and have less pain in the summer? This is not because of the heat but because of the amount of vitamin D created in your body.

....

VITAMIN D REDUCES BREAST CANCER RISK BY 60 PERCENT

Many studies have shown that vitamin D plays a protective role in all kinds of cancers, including breast cancer. A 2007 study of 1,179 women in Nebraska found that postmenopausal women have a 60 percent lower chance of getting cancer if taking vitamin D and calcium supplements.[5] (The study looked at supplementation of both vitamin D and calcium, because it also examined the risk of bone fractures.) Nebraska is at the same latitude as Rome. The results would probably be even worse for Dutch and Belgian women. Many studies suggest that there is a relationship between a lack of vitamin D and various types of cancer. There's increasing evidence for a link between no fewer than 17 types of cancer and vitamin D.[6]

VITAMIN D PROTECTS AGAINST CHRONIC DISEASES

An 11-year study of 30,000 women between 55 and 70 showed that vitamin D, both dietary and in supplements, reduced the risk of rheumatoid arthritis by 28 to 34 percent depending on the amount of intake.[7]

Many degenerative chronic diseases may be related to a vitamin D deficiency. Vitamin D probably also protects against cardiovascular diseases, depression, and type 2 diabetes. It is not for nothing that vitamin D experts worldwide call for a daily intake of 50 mg, or 2,000 IU (international units), of vitamin D by people who live in a moderate climate zone.

Magnesium: Your Energy Transporter

Magnesium is one of the mineral salts that your body cannot create itself and that you must get through diet or supplements. If you're under a lot of stress, be aware that your body, through urination, excretes four times more magnesium than normal. Magnesium is an important supplement during stressful times. If you consume a lot of dairy, coffee, alcohol, or soft drinks, you will also lose a lot of magnesium.

MAGNESIUM IS ESSENTIAL FOR ALL ENZYMES AND HORMONES

Magnesium is needed for the functioning of hundreds of different enzymes in your body that produce, transport, store, and use energy. It ensures the conversion of nutrients in your body into energy. Magnesium is also very important for the proper functioning and relaxation of your muscles and nerves, because it allows for the transfer of the electrical signals (nerve impulses) through the miles of nerves in your body. Muscle cramps are often a signal that you have a magnesium deficiency. Magnesium also helps in hormone production and can therefore contribute to a better hormone balance.

YOUR SKIN CAN ABSORB MAGNESIUM

Your skin can absorb magnesium well. Instead of popping pills, you can apply a magnesium gel or have a bath or footbath with magnesium flakes: both are natural ways to absorb magnesium. If you do take a magnesium supplement, then take about 500 mg per day. Magnesium helps you relax, so take it at night before bed. If you often sleep badly, take a hot bath with magnesium flakes and a calming oil such as lavender and roll into bed. Chances are you'll sleep like a baby.

Omega-3 Fatty Acids:
The Ultimate Anti-inflammatory

You have already read how important omega-3s are for your health. Normally, you should be able to get enough omega-3 fatty acids from your diet. There's plenty in wild oily fish, meat from animals that eat grass, walnuts, hemp seeds, chia seed, flaxseed, and some other healthy oil and fats. Eating oily fish twice a week along with a variety of seeds and nuts should be enough. But what if you don't want to eat that much fish, if any?

FISH OIL

If you don't like fish, you can take a fish oil supplement. However, if you have environmental or animal welfare reasons not to eat too much fish, you won't be happy with fish oil supplements. It turns out that to create one pound of fish oil, 20 pounds of oily fish is needed. If you worry about the overfishing of our oceans, as I do, fish oil is not the solution. In addition, fish are contaminated with mercury. A lot of (cheap) fish oil supplements are not free of this. There is also the risk that fish oil has oxidized during the production process. If you do choose fish oil, find a reliable manufacturer. Fortunately, there are good alternatives.

ALGAL OIL AND KRILL OIL

Fish get omega-3 from the algae and seaweed they eat. So obviously we too can go to the source itself. Eat seaweed where you can, and use algae as a supplement. Excellent sources of algae in supplements are spirulina, chlorella, and marine phytoplankton. You can also choose krill oil (krill is a collective name for small, shrimplike marine animals) or a totally vegan algal oil. The orthomolecular recommendation for the amount of DHA and EPA is 500 to 1,000 mg per day. Usually two capsules are enough.

REMEMBER THIS

- Eat unprocessed foods and stay away from artificial and overly processed foods, and your natural feeling of fullness will return by itself.
- Even healthy foods should not fill more than 80 percent of your stomach.
- Eat the widest possible variety of healthy foods; eat all the colors of the rainbow.
- Superfoods can be a valuable addition; variety is also important with superfoods.
- See supplements as food, but don't just swallow anything.
- Start with a basic supplement. If you think more is needed, first consult with a good orthomolecular physician or therapist.

TOTALLY GREEN
FROZEN BANANA DESSERT

I won't let you go before you've tried my Totally Green Frozen Banana Dessert! It's truly irresistible. I sometimes eat a bowl after a solid workout. Bananas contain potassium—good for a healthy blood pressure—and serotonin, which can reduce your cravings for sweet food.

Peel a ripe banana and cut it into pieces. Put the pieces in a bowl and put it in the freezer, so you always have frozen banana in the freezer. It's also useful for giving a green smoothie just a little bit more flavor.

If you, like me, use spirulina and chlorella in tablet form, grind about 6 tablets in a mortar until you have a fine powder. You can use just chlorella for a nice grass green. If you use just spirulina, the color will be blue green.

Here's What You Need (for 2 servings)
about 20 pieces frozen banana (about 1 banana)
½ cup plant-based milk
1 teaspoon chlorella and/or spirulina powder
grated coconut (for garnish)

Here's How You Make It
Put the frozen banana in your blender or food processor. Let thaw for 5 to 10 minutes. Then add the milk and the green powder, and blend until it's totally green and creamy. Scrape around the edges if necessary. If it's too soft, put it back in the freezer briefly. Serve in a nice glass and sprinkle with grated coconut.

DO YOU HAVE A LANDSCAPE OF LONGING?

Y OU PROBABLY BOUGHT this book out of a desire to change
something in your life. Maybe you want to have more energy;
you might want to get rid of some physical symptoms, or you
might want to you reach a healthy weight. Perhaps all three.

Diet and lifestyle are hard to change: we're often stuck in old habits. I told you in Chapter 5 about how it's good and healthy to change
your diet in small steps and to take your time. We live in a world in
which everything is fast. We can get from New York to Los Ange-
les in six hours. Technology makes life faster, but your body is and
will remain a slow organism. If you decide to learn to play the piano,
you won't be able to play Rachmaninoff's Piano Concerto no. 2 in a
month. Allow yourself time to make a new diet your own. Take a year
to do it. Reorganize your kitchen, buy new ingredients, and maybe
every now and then pick up a new small appliance. Create new
dishes. Every new, easy-to-make, healthy recipe in your repertoire
that you like is an achievement, and each time you find one, it gets
easier. Your taste buds and body will help you with this. But there's

still one more thing that can help you change your eating habits permanently. That is having what I call a "landscape of longing."

WOULD YOU LIKE TO BE RID OF SOMETHING OR TO GO SOMEWHERE?

It is often said that there are two ways to get a stubborn donkey running: you can give it a tap on its butt with a stick or you can offer it a delicious carrot. This also applies to people. In other words, you are spurred into motion only by either something you don't like or the desire to get somewhere that seems much better. Give yourself a minute to remember why you picked up this book: Do you want to leave something behind, or do you want to go somewhere? My experience is that many women are driven by pain: a desire to rid themselves of something—lack of energy, symptoms, or too much weight. If this sounds familiar to you, then I have bad news: the stick does not work. Maybe a little, but never for long. Not with animals, not with children, and not with adult women either.

OLD HABITS PULL YOU BACK TO YOUR OLD WORLD

Pain is the wrong motivation to begin to take action. If you want to stay in forward motion, if you want to go on a voyage, then you need a purpose: a beautiful dream or a landscape you long to be in. You have to put something powerful in front of stubborn old habits that continue to pull you down. Wanting to leave them behind is not enough.

Let's say you want to lose 20 pounds but you have no idea where you want to go—how your life there will look, how you will feel, what you will do, or how you will behave once those 20 pounds are gone. You don't have something you're living for; you don't have a clear goal shining before your eyes. Maybe you're even doing someone else a favor instead of doing it for yourself.

You might lose the first 5 pounds reasonably easily, but as it becomes more difficult and more willpower is required, the urgency is smaller. The pain of being 20 pounds overweight has decreased. You're a clothing size smaller, too, and people may tell you you look good. As soon as it becomes more difficult and the pain is less, old habits pull at you harder than new ones.

Think of it as like a rubber band. You're going up the road with the elastic around your waist, but it's getting harder to stay moving forward on that road because the elastic pulls you back ever harder. Over time you fall back. You give up until the pain is so great that you try going up the road again. This pattern can continue to repeat itself for the rest of your life. A landscape of longing, however, will pull at you like a magnet and makes it easier for you.

WHAT'S YOUR LANDSCAPE OF LONGING?

A landscape of longing can be anything. Maybe you want a better job or a new love affair, or to run a marathon. Maybe you want to feel better, or to have a sense of your own power so that you have an easier time saying no and can stand up for yourself better. You might want to have energy to volunteer, start your own business, or take a trip around the world. What does your dream life look like about a year from now? What makes your heart beat faster, and what makes you excited and happy when you think about it?

Write your longings in a journal or make it a vision board: find images of your ideal life and stick them on a large sheet of bristol board around a picture of yourself. I do it every year in January. Visualization also works powerfully. Successful business people and elite athletes visualize their goals, and for good reason: it makes your subconscious and all the cells in your body aware of where you want to go, and that makes it easier to reach your goals. Trust me, your life is influenced by your subconscious more than you think. Suppose the Universe guaranteed you that you will become a super healthy, creative, happy, and vital 85-year-old. What are you going to do today?

What choices will you make? What do you still want to learn, discover, or experience? What are you good at and what do you enjoy that you want to strengthen and develop?

....
Daydreaming helps you figure out
what's important to you.
....

BE PREPARED TO CHANGE

You belong to the first generation of women who, on their 45th birthday, are only at the halfway point, women who still have an average of 40 years ahead of them. With a bit of luck those will be 40 healthy years, because 80 percent of all diseases in the Western world can be prevented or cured using a healthy diet and a healthy lifestyle. Have faith that if you change your diet, you will find that you change with it. With nutrition, you will change your life. Let go of old ideas about yourself; see curiosity as healthy and toss the words "That's just how I am" into the trash. Be prepared to change—then miracles can happen. I never thought I would have the guts to quit my regular job and start my own business. I had a lifelong hatred of the gym; now I go twice a week and enjoy it. I had always thought that my health would decline after my 40th. I have never felt so healthy, energetic, brave, and powerful as I feel now, well into my 50s, and I know I can do more.

....
The biggest secret of healthy and vital
aging for women is the willingness to change.
....

Get rid of the idea that once you're over 40, your health will deteriorate; that is information from an old world that is disappearing. You're at the wheel of your life and you decide. You have the power to change your life into what you want it to be. It doesn't matter where you come from or where you are now. Dream great dreams, create a landscape of longing that will pull you forward like a magnet, and get on the road full of curiosity. A fantastic life is one in which you let the best of yourself out and allow it to flourish. Change your diet, change your hormones, change your life. The best is yet to come. I promise you.

....

Change your diet, change your hormones, change your life. The best is yet to come. I promise you.

....

SUBSTITUTIONS

Replace This...	...with That
Plain tap water, spring water in plastic bottles	Filtered tap water, spring water in glass bottles
Iodized table salt	Celtic Sea salt, Himalayan salt, tamari
Products packed in tins or plastic	Products packaged in glass or from the freezer (in moderation; note added sugars and other additives)
Sandwich fillings (meat, cheese, sweet spreads)	Homemade spreads based on avocados, hummus, eggs, and/or nuts and vegetables
"Light" products	Non-light versions (in moderation)
Ready-to-use spice mixes and flavor enhancers	A blend of dried or fresh herbs and spices without additives

Replace This...	...with That
Roasted nuts and seeds	Raw nuts and seeds
Roasted peanuts	Raw nuts or, in moderation, raw peanuts
Meat, fish, chicken, and vegetable bouillon cubes	Vegetable bouillon cubes or powder without added yeast extract
Margarine; low-fat margarine	Butter, ghee, or coconut oil
For frying, butter, sunflower oil, corn oil, soybean oil	Coconut oil, red palm oil, or rice germ oil
Corn oil, sunflower oil, ready-made sauces and dressings, mayonnaise, tomato ketchup	Homemade dressings based on extra-virgin olive oil, perilla oil, walnut oil, pumpkin seed oil, flaxseed oil, canola oil, balsamic vinegar, apple cider vinegar, mustard (note additives and sugars)
Nonorganic meat	In moderation: organic meat, chicken, or turkey; organic free-range animals fed natural food
Processed meats (breaded, marinated, seasoned, sausages, burgers, frozen, etc.)	Unprocessed organic meat

Replace This...	...with That
Fish, seafood, shellfish	Plant sources of largely omega-3s (walnuts, hempseed, flaxseed, chia seed, perilla oil); seaweed products (seaweed, salicornia); wild-caught fish; krill oil or algal oil supplements
Animal proteins (dairy, meat, fish)	Vegetable proteins: quinoa, hempseed, vegetables, legumes, tempeh, nuts, seeds, nutritional yeast flakes; spirulina or vegetable protein powder as supplements; milk (and meat) of goat, sheep, or bison (in moderation)
Ready-to-eat meat substitutes	Tempeh, tofu in moderation, and all plant proteins
Nonorganic eggs	Organic eggs
White sugar, synthetic sweeteners and sweeteners, cane syrup, raw cane sugar	In moderation: grade C maple syrup, raw agave syrup, coconut blossom sugar, cold-spun honey, lucuma powder, green stevia powder
Fruit juices, soft drinks, energy drinks, chocolate drinks, soy drinks, and dairy drinks, including all "light" varieties	Water, herbal tea, white tea, green tea, kombucha, coconut water (note additives), fresh-squeezed fruit juice, fruit juice concentrate diluted with five parts water
Cake, candy, ready-to-eat "healthy" candy bars, chocolate	In moderation: homemade cookies or sweets, chocolate (70 percent cocoa or higher)

Replace This...	...with That
White wheat flour, spelt	A mix of gluten-free flours such as buckwheat flour, nut flour, oat flour, seed flour, coconut flour, almond flour, chickpea (gram) flour, quinoa flour, teff flour
Potatoes, mashed potatoes	Sweet potatoes, Jerusalem artichoke, mashed sweet potatoes, pumpkin, celeriac, legumes
White rice	Quinoa, black rice, wild rice, amaranth, cañihua, brown rice in moderation
Milk, buttermilk	Homemade vegetable milk from nuts, seeds, oats, or brown rice
Bread, rusks, crackers, toasts, all made from wheat or spelt	In moderation: sourdough spelt bread, yam dough bread, homemade gluten-free bread, vegetable bread, rice cakes, buckwheat waffles
Pasta made from wheat, spelt, or kamut	Pasta made from buckwheat, quinoa, kelp, or vegetables
Cornstarch, gelatin, unspecified "thickener"	Agar, arrowroot, locust bean gum, buckwheat flour, flaxseed (psyllium)
Yeast	Baking powder, baking soda (sodium bicarbonate) with lemon juice or vinegar

NOTES

Chapter 1. Women Really Are Different

1. R.A. Seguin, C.D. Economos, R. Palombo, R. Hyatt, J. Kuder, and M.E. Nelson, Strength training and older women: A cross-sectional study examining factors related to exercise adherence, *Journal of Aging and Physical Activity* 18(2010):201–18, https://www.ncbi.nlm.nih.gov/pmc/articles/PMC4308058/.

Chapter 2. Work Wisely with Your Hormones

1. P.S. Cooke and A. Naaz, Role of estrogens in adipocyte development and function, *Experimental Biology and Medicine* 229(2004):1127–35.
2. N.A. Brooks, G. Wilcox, K.Z. Walker, J.F. Ashton, M.B. Cox, and L. Stojanovska, Beneficial effects of *Lepidium meyenii* (maca) on psychological symptoms and measures of sexual dysfunction in postmenopausal women are not related to estrogen or androgen content, *Menopause* 15(2008):1157–62, doi: 10.1097/gme.0b013e3181732953.
3. J.A. McLachlan, E. Simpson, and M. Martin, Endocrine disrupters and female reproductive health, *Best Practice & Research: Clinical Endocrinology & Metabolism* 20(2006):63–75.
4. M. de Lorgeril and P. Salen, Helping women to good health: Breast cancer, omega-3/omega-6 lipids, and related lifestyle factors, BMC *Medicine* 12(March 27, 2014), doi: 10.1186/1741-7015-12-54; K.C. Knower, S.Q. To, Y.K. Leung, S.M. Ho, and C.D. Clyne, Endocrine disruption of the epigenome: A breast cancer

link, *Endocrine-Related Cancer* 21 (April 2014):T33–T55, doi: 10.1530/ERC-13-0513; H. Rochefort [Bisphenol A and hormone-dependent cancers: Potential risk and mechanism], *Médecine/sciences* 29(2013):539–44, doi: 10.1051/medsci/2013295019; L. Hilakivi-Clarke, S. de Assis, and A. Warri, Exposures to synthetic estrogens at different times during the life, and their effect on breast cancer risk, *Journal of Mammary Gland Biology and Neoplasia* 18(2013):25–42, doi: 10.1007/s10911-013-9274-8.

5. C. Lauritzen, H.D. Reuter, R. Repges, K.J. Böhnert, and U. Schmidt, Treatment of premenstrual tension syndrome with Vitex agnus castus controlled, double-blind study versus pyridoxine, *Phytomedicine* 4(1997):183–89, doi: 10.1016/S0944-7113(97):80066–69.

6. D.H. Lee, I.K. Lee, K. Song, M. Steffes, W. Toscano, B.A. Baker, and D.R. Jacobs Jr., A strong dose–response relation between serum concentrations of persistent organic pollutants and diabetes: Results from the National Health and Examination Survey 1999–2002, *Diabetes Care* 29(2006):1638–44, doi: 10.2337/dc06-0543.

7. K.W. Taylor, R.F. Novak, H.A. Anderson, L.S. Birnbaum, C. Blystone, M. Devito, … and L. Lind, Evaluation of the association between persistent organic pollutants (POPs) and diabetes in epidemiological studies: A national toxicology program workshop review, *Environmental Health Perspectives* 121(2013): 774–83, doi: 10.1289/ehp.1205502.

8. American Psychological Association, *Stress by gender: A stressful imbalance*, https://www.apa.org/news/press/releases/stress/2012/gender-report.pdf.

9. L.K. Tamres, D. Janicki, and V.S. Helgeson, Sex differences in coping behavior: A meta-analytic review and an examination of relative coping, *Personality and Social Psychology Review* 6(2002):2–30, doi: 10.1207/S15327957PSPR0601_I.

10. P. Methlie, E.E. Husebye, S. Hustad, E.A. Lien, and K. Løvås, Grapefruit juice and licorice increase cortisol availability in patients with Addison's disease, *European Journal of Endocrinology* 165(2011):761–69, doi: 10.1530/EJE-11-0518.

11. E. Diamanti-Kandarakis, J.P. Bourguinon, L.C. Giodice, R. Hauser, G.S. Prins, A.M. Soto, … and A.C. Gore, Endocrine-disrupting chemicals: An Endocrine Society scientific statement, *Endocrine Reviews* 30(2009):293–342, doi: 10.1210/er.2009-0002.

12. Diamanti-Kandarakis et al., Endocrine-disrupting chemicals; C. Sategna-Gui-detti, U. Volta, C. Ciacci, P. Usai, A. Carlino, L. De Franceschi,... and C. Brossa, Prevalence of thyroid disorders in untreated adult celiac disease patients and effect of gluten withdrawal: An Italian multicenter study, American Journal of Gastroenterology 96(2001):751–57, doi: 10.1111/j.1572-0241.2001.03617.x.

13. You can find these here: http://www.ncbi.nlm.nih.gov/pubmed/?term=fluori de+thyroid+function.

14. J.A. Bravo, P. Forsythe, M.V. Chew, E. Escaravage, H.M. Savignac, T.G. Dinan,... and J.F. Cryan, Ingestion of Lactobacillus strain regulates emotional behavior and central GABA receptor expression in a mouse via the vagus nerve, PNAS 108(2011):16050–55, doi: 10.1073/pnas.1102999108.

Chapter 6. Point 1: Eat and Drink as Nature Provides

1. Joanna Blythman, Swallow This: Serving Up the Food Industry's Darkest Secrets (Fourth Estate, 2015), 191.

2. Kitta MacPherson, Sugar can be addictive, Princeton scientist says, Princeton University press release, December 10, 2008, http://www.princeton.edu/main/news/archive/s22/88/56G31.

3. Michael Moss, Salt Sugar Fat: How the Food Giants Hooked Us (Signal, 2013), xxvii.

4. Moss, xxvi.

5. Zorg over kwaliteit van bronnen voor drinkwater, April 4, 2013, Rijksinsti-tuut voor Volksgezondheid en Milieu, http://www.rivm.nl/Documenten _en_publicaties/Algemeen_Actueel/Nieuwsberichten/2013/Zorg_over _kwaliteit_van_bronnen_voor_drinkwater; Nederlands Drinkwaterbesluit, November 28, 2015, http://wetten.overheid.nl/BWBR0030111/2015-11-28; Inspectie Leefomgeving en ransport, Ministerie van Infrastructuur en Milieu, Kwaliteit van het Nederlands drinkwater in 2014, November 5, 2015, https://www.rijksoverheid.nl/binaries/rijksoverheid/documenten/rapporten /2015/11/24/ilt-rapport-de-kwaliteit-van-het-drinkwater-in-nederland-in-2014/ilt-rapport-de-kwaliteit-van-het-drinkwater-in-nederland-in-2014.pdf.

Chapter 7. Point 2: Don't Fear Healthy Fats (and Eat Them!)

1. For the Nurses' Health Study, see http://www.nhs3.org/index.php/about-us; for the Women's Health Initiative, see https://www.nhlbi.nih.gov/whi/

background.htm. For studies, see, for example, B. Forette, D. Tortrat, and Y. Wolmark, Cholesterol as risk factor for mortality in elderly women, *The Lancet* (April 22, 1989):868–70.

2. B. Goldman, Osteoarthritis results from inflammatory process, not just wear and tear, study suggests, Stanford Medicine News Center (November 6, 2011), http://med.stanford.edu/news/all-news/2011/11/osteoarthritis-results-from-inflammatory-process-not-just-wear-and-tear-study-suggests.html.

Chapter 8. Point 3: Eat an Abundance of Vegetables

1. World Cancer Research Fund International, *Second Expert Report* (2007), http://www.wcrf.org/int/research-we-fund/continuous-update-project-cup/second-expert-report.

2. R. Béliveau and D. Gingras, *Eten tegen kanker* (Kosmos Uitgevers, 2016).

3. C.B. Esselstyn Jr., S.G. Ellis, S.V. Medendorp, and T.D. Crowe, A strategy to arrest and reverse coronary artery disease: A 5-year longitudinal study of a single physician's practice, *Journal of Family Practice* 41(1995):560–68.

4. E. Cho, W.Y. Chen, D.J. Hunter, M.J. Stampfer, G.A. Colditz, S.E. Hankinson, and W.C. Willett, Red meat intake and risk of breast cancer among premenopausal women, *Archives of Internal Medicine* 166(2006):2253–59, doi: 10.1001/archinte.166.20.2253.

5. E. Krieger, L.D. Youngman, and T.C. Campbell, The modulation of aflatoxin (AFB1) induced preneoplastic lesions by dietary protein and voluntary exercise in Fischer 344 rats, *Nutrition and Cancer* 2(1992):131–42, doi: 10.1080/01635589209514213.

Chapter 9. Point 4: Be Smarter Than Sweets

1. P. Pedram, D. Wadden, P. Amini, W. Gulliver, E. Randell, F. Cahill, ... and G. Sun, Food addiction: Its prevalence and significant association with obesity in the general population, PLOS ONE 8(2013):e74832, doi: 10.1371/journal.pone.0074832.

2. S.E. Racine, K.M. Culbert, P.K. Keel, C.L. Sisk, S.A. Burt, and K.L. Klump, Differential associations between ovarian hormones and disordered eating symptoms across the menstrual cycle in women, *International Journal of Eating Disorders* (June 7, 2011), doi: 10.1002/eat.20941.

3. M. Lenoir, F. Serre, L. Cantin, and S.H. Ahmed, Intense sweetness surpasses cocaine reward, PLOS ONE One 2(2007):e698, doi: 10.1371/journal.pone.0000698.

4. G. Fagherazzi, A. Vilier, D.S. Sartorelli, M. Lajous, B. Balkau, and F. Clavel-Chapelon, Consumption of artificially and sugar-sweetened beverages and incident type 2 diabetes in the Etude Epidémiologique auprès des femmes de la Mutuelle Générale de l'Education Nationale–European Prospective Investigation into Cancer and Nutrition cohort, *American Journal of Clinical Nutrition* 97(2013):517–23, doi: 10.3945/ajcn.112.050997.

5. S.E. Swithers and T.L. Davidson, A role for sweet taste: Calorie predictive relations in energy regulation by rats, *Behavioral Neuroscience* 122(2008):161–73, doi: 10.1037/0735-7044.122.1.161.

6. Tina Thomas, *Who Do You Think You Are? Understanding Your Personality from the Inside Out* (Morgan James, 2016).

Chapter 10. Point 5: Cow's Milk Is for Calves

1. D. Feskanich, W.C. Willett, M.J. Stampfer, and G.A. Colditz, Milk, dietary calcium, and bone fractures in women: A 12-year prospective study, *American Journal of Public Health* 87(1997):992–97.

2. K. Fairfield, Annual Meeting of the Society for General Internal Medicine: Dairy products linked to ovarian cancer risk, *Family Practice News* (June 11, 2000).

Chapter 11. Point 6: Intestines Do Not Like Gluten

1. R. Kuipers, *Het oerdieet: de manier om oergezond oud te worden* (Taschenbuch, 2013).

2. William Davis, *Wheat Belly: Lose the Wheat, Lose the Weight, and Find Your Path Back to Health* (Rodale, 2011), 50.

3. David Perlmutter, *Grain Brain: The Surprising Truth about Wheat, Carbs, and Sugar—Your Brain's Silent Killers* (Little, Brown, 2013), 61.

4. A.L. Culver, I.S. Ockene, R. Balasubramanian, B.C. Olendzki, D.M. Sepavich, J. Wactawski-Wende, ... and Y. Ma, Statin use and risk of diabetes mellitus in postmenopausal women in the Women's Health Initiative, *Archives of Internal Medicine* 172(2012):144–52, doi: 10.1001/archinternmed.2011.625.

5. S. Seneff, How statins really work explains why they don't really work (2011), https://people.csail.mit.edu/seneff/why_statins_dont_really_work.html.

Chapter 12. Point 7: Eat Many Different Things (but Don't Eat Too Much)

1. Michael Pollan, In Defense of Food: An Eater's Manifesto (Penguin, 2008).
2. Christiane Northrup, The Wisdom of Menopause (Bantam, 2012).
3. A Consortium of Scientists, Institutions and Individuals Committed to Solving the Worldwide Vitamin D Deficiency Epidemic, Scientists' call to D*action: The vitamin D deficiency epidemic, revised (Grassroots Health, 2015), https://grassrootshealth.net/wp-content/uploads/2016/11/scientists _call_to_daction_020113.pdf.
4. P. Christiaans and H. Roskamp, De houdbare vrouw: praktische gids voor een eeu-wige jeugd (CocoBooks, 2009), 107.
5. J.M. Lappe, D. Travers-Gustafson, K.M. Davies, R.R. Recker, and R.P. Heaney, Vitamin D and calcium supplementation reduces cancer risk: Results of a randomized trial, American Journal of Clinical Nutrition 85(2007):1586–91.
6. W.B. Grant, C.F. Garland, and E.D. Gorham, An estimate of cancer mortality rate reductions in Europe and the US with 1,000 IU of oral vitamin D per day, Recent Results in Cancer Research 174(2007):225–34.
7. L.A. Merlino, J. Curtis, T.R. Mikuls, J.R. Cerhan, L.A. Criswell, K.G. Saag, and Iowa Women's Health Study, Vitamin D intake is inversely associated with rheumatoid arthritis: Results from the Iowa Women's Health Study, Arthritis and Rheumatism 50(2004):72–77, doi: 10.1002/art.11434.

ACKNOWLEDGMENTS

Thank you so much!

YOU NEVER WRITE a book alone—so many people have helped me. Thanks to all the writers whose books and articles I have devoured over the past few years. You don't know me, but I've learned so much from you: Ruth Heidrich, Sara Gottfried, Christiane Northrup, Amy Myers, Michael Moss, Mark Hyman, and many, many others.

Thanks Miriam, Astrid, and Barbara for reading earlier versions of the manuscript and for your valuable advice and comments.

Thank you, above all, Hester, for all your professional additions and rigorous editorial work. It was a pleasure to be able to work together with you.

Thank you so much once again, Ralph and Barbara, for all I've learned from you. Without knowing it, you have stood at the cradle of this book.

Thanks, Sue, Anouschka, Saskia, Yolande, Michelle, Inge, and Tanja for your inspiring enthusiasm and creativity around the original final design of this book. I have enjoyed working with all of you!

Thank you, Martine, Maaike, Willemijn, Suzanne, and Jan van Cosmos for your enthusiasm and trust in this book and for your dedication.

Thank you so much, Rob, for all the hours we sparred about this book, long before there was a word on the page; you will recognize many of our conversations here.

But above all, many thanks to all my loyal newsletter readers who have waited patiently until this book finally saw the light of day. This book certainly would not exist without you. You are the wind beneath my wings!

INDEX